The *Sexy Little Book* of

ORAL
PLEASURE

Ava Cadell, Ph.D., Ed.D.

ALPHA

A member of Penguin Group (USA) Inc.

ALPHA BOOKS

Published by Penguin Group (USA) Inc.

Penguin Group (USA) Inc., 375 Hudson Street, New York, New York 10014, USA • Penguin Group (Canada), 90 Eglinton Avenue East, Suite 700, Toronto, Ontario M4P 2Y3, Canada (a division of Pearson Penguin Canada Inc.) • Penguin Books Ltd., 80 Strand, London WC2R 0RL, England • Penguin Ireland, 25 St. Stephen's Green, Dublin 2, Ireland (a division of Penguin Books Ltd.) • Penguin Group (Australia), 250 Camberwell Road, Camberwell, Victoria 3124, Australia (a division of Pearson Australia Group Pty. Ltd.) • Penguin Books India Pvt. Ltd., 11 Community Centre, Panchsheel Park, New Delhi—110 017, India • Penguin Group (NZ), 67 Apollo Drive, Rosedale, North Shore, Auckland 1311, New Zealand (a division of Pearson New Zealand Ltd.) • Penguin Books (South Africa) (Pty.) Ltd., 24 Sturdee Avenue, Rosebank, Johannesburg 2196, South Africa • Penguin Books Ltd., Registered Offices: 80 Strand, London WC2R 0RL, England

International Standard Book Number: 978-1-61564-134-5
Library of Congress Catalog Card Number: 2011904915

16   15   14   8   7   6   5   4   3

Interpretation of the printing code: The rightmost number of the first series of numbers is the year of the book's printing; the rightmost number of the second series of numbers is the number of the book's printing. For example, a printing code of 11-1 shows that the first printing occurred in 2011.

Printed in the United States of America

Note: This publication contains the opinions and ideas of its author. It is intended to provide helpful and informative material on the subject matter covered. It is sold with the understanding that the author and publisher are not engaged in rendering professional services in the book. If the reader requires personal assistance or advice, a competent professional should be consulted.

The author and publisher specifically disclaim any responsibility for any liability, loss, or risk, personal or otherwise, which is incurred as a consequence, directly or indirectly, of the use and application of any of the contents of this book.

Trademarks: All terms mentioned in this book that are known to be or are suspected of being trademarks or service marks have been appropriately capitalized. Alpha Books and Penguin Group (USA) Inc. cannot attest to the accuracy of this information. Use of a term in this book should not be regarded as affecting the validity of any trademark or service mark.

Most Alpha books are available at special quantity discounts for bulk purchases for sales promotions, premiums, fund-raising, or educational use. Special books, or book excerpts, can also be created to fit specific needs.

For details, write: Special Markets, Alpha Books, 375 Hudson Street, New York, NY 10014.

This book is dedicated to my husband, Peter Knecht,
"The Cunnilingus Guru."

Contents

Contents

Introduction

First I'd like to congratulate you for picking up *The Sexy Little Book of Oral Pleasure.* This book is for busy, adventurous people who want no-holds-barred, straight-to-the-point information on titillating, erotic, and luscious oral sex for men and women.

I have written this book so it will be fun and easy to find whatever question, technique, or fact you are looking for. It offers an expansion of your oral sex horizon including detailed information about stimulating various male and female pleasure spots, advanced oral sex positions, and how to achieve the ultimate orgasm, a TriGasm. It will help you to avoid oral pitfalls and even teach you the latest slang words for oral sex and your genitals.

Whether you are an oral sex virgin or an oral sex master, this book will be a valuable tool to ensure that you have the best oral sex experience possible, making every oral sex encounter a memorable one. I believe everyone can learn more about oral sex, and can become an outstanding lover. As a leading sex expert, I've been teaching thousands of singles and couples all around the globe how to have healthy sex and relationships for more than a decade. While writing this book, even I learned some new dynamics on oral sex.

Extras

Enjoy extra bits of information and explanations on various oral sex topics and terms throughout the book in these sidebars. They are:

Definitions and significant facts about oral sex, which can also be informative or cautionary.

Insights on the penis or other aspects of male sexuality.

Sex tips for making your oral technique and experience better.

Insights on the vagina and other aspects of female sexuality.

Acknowledgments

Thanks to Mikal E. Belicove, acquisitions editor at Alpha Books for Penguin Group (USA) Inc., for offering me the chance to write this book, and to Nancy Lewis, my editor, whose contributions were excellent and enjoyable. Special gratitude goes to my patient husband, Peter Knecht, who hardly saw me while I was working on this book; to Shelly Barnum, my right hand who managed to juggle running my company and analyzing my book simultaneously; to Kim Yaged, for her resourceful research; and to my stepson, Chance, who is now a master of slang.

1

Oral Sex 101

Let's begin our oral pleasure journey by laying down some basics and key fundamentals about oral sex. In this chapter, we'll explore what exactly oral sex is and what it's called, including slang and common terms. Next, we'll understand why men and women love oral sex so much and why it's an important part of a healthy sex life. Finally, we'll learn about sexual inhibitions you may have, where they come from, and how to get rid of them. This chapter will help you get rid of old, negative attitudes toward oral pleasure and prepare you for a healthy oral sex experience.

Also, in this book, you will find the references to sexual partners and lovers as men and women together. However, the information and techniques provided in this book apply to all partners and lovers, regardless of sexual orientation. Any person and any couple who wants to enhance and expand their knowledge of oral pleasure will benefit from reading this book. You, and your lover, will be glad you did. So let's get started.

What Is Oral Sex?

Oral sex refers to all sexual activities involving the use of the mouth (lips, tongue, throat, or teeth) to sexually lick, kiss, suck, or nibble the male or female genitals. Orally satisfying the sexual organs should be pleasurable to both the giver and the receiver of oral sex. Since the male sexual organs, the female sexual organs, as well as the mouth and tongue are sensitive with lots of nerve endings, of course it should feel good to both partners.

Oral sex can be a prelude to intercourse, it can be the main event, or it can be a form of afterplay, too. The choice is yours and your partner's.

Oral sex can be enjoyed as the receiver, the giver, or both, and the more you trust each other the better your experiences will be. You can receive oral sex selfishly or as a loving gift from your partner. You can give it and be equally aroused as your partner receiving it—women can even reach their own orgasms while giving their lover oral sex. You and your lover can give and receive it simultaneously in a sixty-nine position (more on this in Chapter 9).

Some people engage in oral sex instead of intercourse as a means of contraception (birth control). Oral sex can be used for pleasure even when avoiding pregnancy is not a concern.

Is Oral Sex Really Sex?

In the minds of many teenagers, oral sex isn't really sex. They may think they can stay virgins by engaging in oral sex because a girl's hymen isn't broken. That's like saying you can have anal sex and remain a virgin. Technically, it's true, but theoretically and emotionally it's not. Oral sex is just as intimate as sexual intercourse, so why would you engage in oral sex with someone you wouldn't want to have intercourse with?

Some men even think they aren't cheating when they have oral sex with another woman. The truth is, giving and receiving oral sex is considered one of the most intimate and erotic acts that can be exchanged within a loving adult relationship … and yes, oral sex is sex!

The Various Names

The medical term for oral sex is *irrumation,* which literally means "to suck." The technical term for oral sex performed on a man is *fellatio; cunnilingus* when performed on a woman.

Fellatio comes from the Latin word fellare, meaning "to suck." Fellatio is oral sex performed on a man's penis that may or may not be continued to orgasm and ejaculation. **Cunnilingus** comes from the Latin words cunnus, meaning "vulva," and lingere, meaning "to lick."

A common slang term for giving oral sex to either a man or woman is "giving head." Done on the genitals of a man, common slang is a "blow job," or BJ for short. Done on the genitals of a woman, common slang is "eating her out." For both sexes, the common phrase used is to "go down on someone."

Although it is called giving a man a "blow" job, it is actually accomplished by sucking on the man's penis. The term blow job is believed to stem from eighteenth-century Europe, when prostitutes were called blowers. During the 1930s, prostitutes would offer to blow off their customers. It wasn't until the mid-1960s that the term blow job was commonly used, after a film was released by Andy Warhol titled *Blow Job*. In the film, there were several explicit descriptions of the act.

Most people usually use slang terms when talking about oral sex during sex, and this in itself can be a turn on.

Say the slang words that you find the most erotic and then ask your lover to repeat them. If you tell your lover which words turn you on the most, you can both use them during lovemaking and oral sex.

Slang for Cunnilingus

Over the years, giving oral sex to a woman has had many descriptive slang names ranging from gobbling, yummy it down, eating out, cunt lapping, polishing the pearl, plating, carpet munching, canyon yodeling, eating pussy, muff diving, frenching, alphabetizing, bag lunch, beaver dinner, bird licking, box lunch, fur-burger feast, bush doctor, cherry flip, chewing bubble gum, chow box, clam dinner, and the genital kiss.

Slang for Vagina

Many women are uncomfortable hearing or saying slang words for the vagina like twat, snatch, beaver, clam, slit, or cunt because they think they have negative connotations. Most women are comfortable with the word pussy to describe their vagina, especially when it's used in a compliment like, "Your pussy looks beautiful." In contrast, the ancient Tantric (sacred and spiritual sex teachings) worship for women's genitals is illustrated by a host of lyrical words like Jade Gate, Jade Chamber, and Golden Furrow. The ancient Hindu term yoni has achieved some notoriety today and has more respectful overtones.

Slang for Fellatio

Common slang terms for fellatio include blow job and sucking off. Also, to go down on, give head, 68 (you do me, and I'll owe you one), breathing through the ears, buff the helmet, buff the knob, butterfly flick, checking the mike, choking, chomping the chicken, cleaning your head, hum job, hummer, playing the skin flute, dick licking, and cock sucking.

Slang for Penis (and Testicles)

Men really don't have a problem with calling their penis by slang names. In fact, it turns most men on when a woman calls it a cock, especially if she says, "Your cock looks and feels so good." Other popular terms for the penis include arrow, baloney, woody, beaver cleaver, schlong, beef bayonet, pork sword, lap taffy, pecker, dick, prick, and bishop. Let's not forget about slang words for the testicles, which include balls, nuts, bag, cobblers, goolies, and the boys.

Naming Each Other's Genitals

Men and women also like to name their genitals or give each other's genitals pet names. Here are some popular penis names: Peter, John Thomas, Johnson, Godzilla, Mr. Happy, Long John, Tiger, and the Monster. Women like more sensitive or cute names for their vaginas like lotus, lily, petal, pearl, kitty, cookie, or coochie.

When couples name each other's genitals, they often use famous historical couples like Adam and Eve, Caesar and Cleopatra, Napoleon and Josephine, or Bonnie and Clyde. Couples can have fun talking about their genitals in public and others won't have a clue what they are talking about. For example, a guy might say something like, "How is Cleopatra feeling today?" She could reply, "Cleo would like to get some attention because she's feeling a little neglected." With that, he could answer back, "You tell Cleo that I've come to bury Caesar, not to praise him."

It's all about communicating your wants and needs in a playful manner. Think of sex as adult play, because too many people take sex far too seriously.

What Oral Sex Can Be

It's important to remember that oral sex at its best is a mutual giving and receiving. Here are some examples of what oral sex can be:

- A precious gift to someone who is worthy to receive it. Our sexual gifts are as valuable as any other part of ourselves that we prize. Selecting the right sexual partner to give to and receive from is as important a decision as choosing anything you place a high value on.

- A natural high, perhaps even the best of nature's uplifts. It can energize us and make us feel more creative afterward.

- A wonderful form of self-expression, infinitely artistic. It is both beautiful and erotic. It is gentle and assertive. It is relaxing and energizing.

- A way to renew stamina, not deplete it. It can free us from emotional stress and release any tension and discomfort lodged in our muscles.

But most of all, it is a unique connection between two people who want to share a divine pleasure.

Our Basic Sexual Rights

Our basic human rights extend to include our sexual rights, too. These include the following.

- As adults, we have the right to engage in consensual sex.

- We all have the right to a sex life, including people who are physically and mentally disadvantaged.

- We are free to think of any sexual thought or fantasy.

- We have the right to determine our own sexuality.

- As adults, we are free to choose our own sexual entertainment in the legal marketplace.

- We have the right to not be exposed to unwanted sexual behavior or materials.

For men and women to achieve a full and satisfying sex life, which is each individual's right, they need self-knowledge, facts, techniques, and honesty, all of which are available in this book.

Why Men Love Oral Sex

Men love getting oral sex from a woman because it's like having intercourse in her mouth. Her soft lips wrap around his penis and her wet tongue dances around it as her hot mouth sucks him deeper and deeper—this is the ultimate pleasure for many red-blooded men. In fact, 90.5 percent of men say they love getting oral sex. It's a basic male instinct to seek oral gratification.

When a woman gives a man oral sex, he not only receives physical satisfaction, but he also gets the visual pleasure of watching his lover between his legs. A man feels like he's gone to seventh heaven when his lover orally worships his penis, especially if she's enjoying it. Even though this book is filled with endless oral sex tips and techniques, enthusiasm is still more important than talent.

Men also love oral sex either because it gives him the feeling of being serviced by his lover, which results in a sense of power for him, or he gets gratification from being submissive to his lover while receiving oral sex. These men love to surrender their most precious body part to their lover so she can overpower him with her mouth.

Both the first and second emotions make a man feel accepted and valued by his lover, so there is an emotional and physical connection between them that takes them to a higher level of intimacy. It also makes a man feel confident and gives him high self-esteem, especially sexually.

When you are the receiver of oral sex, try expressing a sexual fantasy that includes you and your partner. Be as graphic as you can; and use words and phrases that turn you both on.

Why Women Love Oral Sex

Although it is more common to hear how men overwhelmingly love oral sex performed on them more than women do, many women out there love oral sex performed on them, too. If, as a woman, you have to ask why, then you have definitely bought the right book.

Some women claim to enjoy oral sex more than sexual inter-course. There is no risk of pregnancy, less chance of catching a sexually transmitted disease (STD), and it's the easiest way for many women to reach a climax. Emotionally, it allows a woman to surrender herself to the pleasure of receiving. Oral sex also helps make a woman feel sexually confident, uninhibited, and worthy.

2

Understanding Her Body

The more you know about a woman's body, the better lover you will be. In this chapter, we'll go on an anatomical journey and discover a woman's sexual body parts. You'll empower yourself by learning the mystery of the female sexual arousal cycle and orgasms, and understanding the delicacy of a woman's vagina. We'll also touch on safer oral sex and supplies.

Her Body Parts

The anatomic variety that makes each person unique is reflected all over our bodies, including our sexual parts. Every woman's breasts and vagina differ in a variety of ways, including color, size, shape, and proportion. So don't expect all boobs and vaginas to look the same, and don't compare them to those of other women, ever.

Welcome and praise all of your lover's parts, because no matter what shape or size they all are, it has no effect on her sexual pleasure and orgasmic ability.

Now let's examine each sensuous part, one by one.

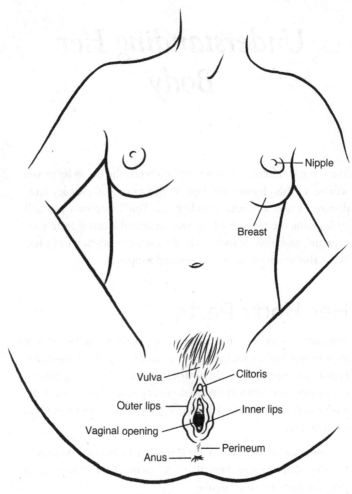

Female sex organs.

The Vulva

The vulva is the visible outer area of the female genitalia, including the pubic hair area (mons veneris). Some women never groom their pubic hair while others style and trim it, bikini-line wax it, or even shave it off completely because they and/or their partner like the way it looks and feels.

The vulva consists of various parts, and when it comes to oral sex, many of these parts are neglected. It's like sitting down to eat a freshly cooked artichoke and abandoning all the leaves to get to the center of the artichoke. It's true that the heart is the tastiest and most tender, but by slowly pulling the petals apart, sucking on each one delicately, you'll create more anticipation, get more nourishment, and still experience devouring the succulent heart of the artichoke.

Did you know that the less pubic hair a woman has, the fewer odors she will have? Another advantage to having a slick vulva is that it's easier to lick, and the extra visual charge can really turn on the partner.

The Vaginal Lips

The first set of vaginal lips are the outer lips (labia majora), which are cushioned with fat and help protect the genitals inside, much like the male scrotum. The outer lips are naturally covered in hair and have a variety of sizes, ranging from small to large, puffy to thin. The texture of the outer lips also differs from smooth to crinkled, and the color of the outer lips can range from pale pink to dark brown. The outer lips may be slightly apart, revealing the inner lips (labia minora), or they may hide the entire area. Licking and sucking the outer lips of a woman's vagina can be extremely pleasurable for her.

The inner lips have no hair or fat filling. They stretch from one end of the vulva to the other, meeting at two corners. At one end they form a protective covering for the clitoris, and at the other end they meet at the *perineum,* the area that separates the vagina from the anus. Rich in nerve endings, the inner lips can result in orgasm when lavished with oral sex because they are connected to the clitoris.

The **perineum** is the area between the anus and vagina in women, and the anus and scrotum in men. A slang term used for perineum is "taint," because it "taint" butt or vagina and it "taint" butt or scrotum. I refer to it affectionately as a "landing strip." Use whatever term works best for you.

The Vaginal Opening

The vaginal opening is the hollow, muscle-lined tube that extends from its opening between a woman's legs up to her cervix, located deep inside the vagina. The vaginal opening connects a woman's external and internal reproductive organs and can expand to many times its normal size (giving birth). It's a real treat for a woman to have her vaginal opening licked and orally penetrated.

The Clitoris

The clitoris is a very important part of the female genitalia when it comes to sex, especially oral sex. Many women find it easier to reach an orgasm while they are receiving oral sex than when they are having sexual intercourse, because most intercourse positions simply don't stimulate the clitoris as directly as a talented tongue can. This is an anatomical fact because the clitoris is located above the vagina, making it difficult for the penis to stimulate it during penetration. The majority of women are able to reach a mind-blowing orgasm by receiving oral sex directly on or around her clitoris.

The clitoris consists of four parts:

- The head (glans), the only visible part of the clitoris.

- The clitoral hood, or the *prepuce,* a protective fold of tissue. The hood can sometimes make it difficult to locate the clitoris. In some women, the clitoral hood has several folds, making it even harder to find.

- The shaft, located below the clitoral head and extends from the head to beneath the hood.

- The crura, two small wings located below the shaft and invisible to the eye.

The clitoris is located at the top of the inner lips, where the lips are joined together.

If you can imagine the vagina as an ice-cream sundae, the clitoris is the cherry on top. When stimulated, the clitoris can grow up to three times its normal size, much like the penis. So it's no surprise that the clitoris is regarded as the female equivalent of the penis and the clitoral hood is equal to the foreskin.

> The clitoris has absolutely no function other than orgasmic pleasure. It has the highest number of concentrated nerve fibers found in the human body—8,000 to be exact. That's higher than anywhere else in the body and twice as many as the man's penis.

The clitoris was designed to open sexual doors for women, literally. The very word *clitoris* derives from the Greek word for key, as in the key to female sexuality. It opens up women to pleasure. The clitoris has its own rhythm and will not be rushed. A woman must have a connection from her brain, and the fantasies it activates, to her clitoris, thereby taking responsibility for her own satisfaction. If her mind is in harmony with her clitoris, she is moving with her own sexual rhythm.

The Anus

The anus is below the vagina at the opposite end of the perineum. The anus is surrounded by sensitive nerve endings making it a source of great pleasure for those daring enough to explore it, and to let it be explored. We will discuss oral stimulation techniques for the anus in detail in Chapter 9.

The G-Spot

The G-spot, for Grafenburg spot, is located deep inside the vagina and cannot be seen, only felt. We will discuss the G-spot in detail later in this chapter since it warrants its own long and all-important explanation. Also, step-by-step instructions on how to find this mysterious and magical spot and how to stimulate it are explained in Chapter 10.

The Breasts

A woman's breasts and nipples are an essential part of her feminine sexuality and her oral sex experience (as well as her partner's). Breasts and nipples, no matter what their size and shape, are full of sensitive nerve endings eager for oral stimulation.

Nipple stimulation in particular promotes the production of the hormones oxytocin and prolactin, which are important for breastfeeding, but also create feelings of bonding, trust, and sexual arousal. Some women can actually achieve orgasm without any other forms of sexual stimulation. Chapter 7 explores this orgasmic potential of the nipples and the techniques you can use to achieve it.

A Healthy Vagina

The vagina is a self-cleaning organ and has a perfect pH balance containing friendly bacteria and lactic acid to keep it healthy and clean. It flushes out dead cells on its own much like our nose dispels mucus when we blow it. To keep it hygienic, do not put anything unsanitary inside it. That includes dirty fingers, a penis that has penetrated the anus, unclean sex toys, foods, and oil-based products (just to name a few). When a woman's pH gets out of balance, her natural secretions smell stronger and she is prone to getting infections. My motto is, "If in doubt, leave it out." Also, a healthy vagina does not need any douching. In fact, douching can change the pH balance of the vagina and cause infections.

The best way for a woman to keep her vagina clean and healthy is to bathe regularly with soap (preferably hypoallergenic soap) and water, pulling back the hood of the clitoris occasionally to clean it with a cotton swab; by checking herself regularly for any changes to her genitals or in her libido, and having annual gynecological check-ups.

Taste and Smell Your Best

One of the most common reasons women don't enjoy receiving oral sex is because they fear their genitals will smell or taste bad. The truth is that a woman's flavor and aroma is influenced by her monthly cycle, diet, medications, vitamins, stress level, and even her environment. As you might expect, if you eat healthfully, drink plenty of water, and keep your stress level down to a minimum, you'll taste your best. The natural taste of a woman's vagina can span from slightly sweet, salty, tangy, to even a trace of iron around the time of her menstrual cycle.

If you haven't already, smell and taste your own sexual juices. To enjoy oral sex, you have to enjoy your own sex organs—this means appreciating everything about them.

Plenty of people find the natural body aromas much more arousing than the reek of pungent perfumes and intimate body sprays. Our sense of smell is the strongest factor in sexual attraction. There's nothing dirty or unpleasant about genital odors and secretions (except in the case of certain vaginal infections, which can result in an unpleasant odor).

If you feel that a little body odor goes a long way, you might be more comfortable taking a shower or bath, or sponge-bathing each other before oral sex. When it comes to oral sex, cleanliness equals confidence.

Her Stages of Sexual Arousal

Human sexuality researchers William Masters and Virginia Johnson conducted the first groundbreaking study of the sexual response cycle in St. Louis in the 1960s, when they studied more than 10,000 sexual response cycles. Their findings described the sexual response cycle as having four stages: excitement, plateau, orgasm, and resolution. I believe there are actually five stages in the cycle for a woman, with the first being foreplay. Let's explore each stage.

Stage #1: Foreplay. Most women need to be prepared for sex with some foreplay. One method is whispering her name in her ear and then kissing her to release pleasure endorphins that will flood her brain with feel-good hormones like serotonin and dopamine. Blood flow will increase to her genitals, and her body will become sensitive all over. Now she's ready for the next stage of sexual arousal.

Stage #2: Excitement. Sexual excitement affects the entire body with the increase of her heart, pulse, and respiration rates. During this cycle, her breasts swell and her nipples become erect. Also, her vagina becomes wet and her clitoris grows up to three times its normal size.

Stage #3: Plateau. Her body temperature rises and changes the color of her inner vaginal lips to a deep red. Her clitoris retracts under the clitoral hood. Her uterus pulls upward into the abdomen, widening the vaginal space and allowing the penis to fit comfortably.

Stage #4: Orgasm. In the orgasm cycle, the uterus, anus, leg muscles, face, and hands begin to involuntarily contract. There are strong contractions in the vagina at 0.8 second intervals, 40 breaths per minute, and a heart rate that can go as high as 180 beats per minute.

Stage #5: Resolution. Cooling down is defined by how long it takes for a woman to get her pulse rate back down to normal and let the rush of blood to her pelvis subside. Blood pressure and pulse gradually return to pre-arousal levels. Swelling in the genitals and other areas decreases. The inner vaginal lips return to their normal color. Muscles relax, and organs and tissues resume their original positions.

During the resolution cycle, stay with your partner and hold her close. This physical connection after oral sex or any other kind of sex is most significant for a woman. It makes her feel like you care about her.

Orgasms vary between women and for the same woman at different times. There is no right or wrong kind of orgasm. Feelings will vary with kind and degree of stimulation, but also with how the woman feels about herself, her partner, and their relationship. Orgasms are described in many different ways but, in common, there is a sensation of building "pressure" or "tension" followed by a sense of inevitability once it starts and "relief" or "release" when it's finished. We'll explore orgasms in more detail in Chapter 7.

Better She Be Safe Than Sorry

If you love yourself, you must protect yourself. There's no reason why women can't enjoy the eroticism of oral sex and practice safer sex at the same time. Even if you're in a monogamous relationship, you'll want to have some of the safer sex supplies around to help you add more pleasure, diversity, and spontaneity to your oral sex adventures.

Along with the information that follows, also see Chapter 3 for information on safer sex for men, including condoms and lubricants.

Female Condoms

Female condoms are soft, loose-fitting sheaths specifically designed to protect women from pregnancy and STDs by lining the inside of her vagina. They're made of polyurethane (stronger than latex) and are hypoallergenic, heat conductive, and odorless. Female condoms are also called FC Female Condoms, and popular brand names include Reality Condoms and Femidom. Read the instructions before inserting a female condom because if you don't insert it correctly, it's like not using protection at all. The female condom has to go deep inside the vagina and over the cervix.

Dental Dams

Aptly named because they are used by dentists to isolate a tooth to be worked on, dental dams are also used for safer oral sex. Available in various sizes and flavors, dental dams are latex, square-shape barriers that allow good sensations for oral sex. Sheer Glyde Dams are FDA (Food and Drug Administration) approved for protection against STDs for cunnilingus and rimming (anal oral sex).

The best way to use a dam is for the giver to mark his "mouth" side of the dam so he knows which side he's going to lick, then apply a couple drops of lubricant on the other side, press the dam against her vagina with two hands, and enjoy.

Latex Gloves and Finger Cots

Good oral sex involves the hands as well as the mouth. There's nothing more exciting than orally pleasing a woman's clitoris and fingering her vagina or anus simultaneously. By using latex gloves and finger cots (think of them as mini-condoms for your fingers), you can increase erotic sensations and protect the receiver from jagged fingernails, cuts, germs, or viral STDs such as herpes, which can be spread by skin-to-skin contact.

⟨ Have fun! ⟩

3

Understanding His Body

Now let's explore the intricacies of the male sexual anatomy and all its pleasurable parts. In this chapter, you'll get to know all the parts of the penis, testicles, and anus. You'll also learn about his sexual arousal cycle, as well as what condoms are best for oral sex and how to tell if your lover has an STD.

His Body Parts

All men are concerned about the size and appearance of their penis, and every guy knows exactly how long his erection is. The average length of a man's erect penis in the United States is 5.1 inches.

If you're wondering how that size compares to the rest of the world, consider that America is a melting pot of many nations and races, so in our country, we run the gamut of small, medium, and large penis sizes, with the average length being 5.1 inches. Remember that the most sensitive part on a woman is her clitoris and the first two inches inside her vagina, so if a penis is two inches or more, there's no reason why it can't satisfy a woman sexually.

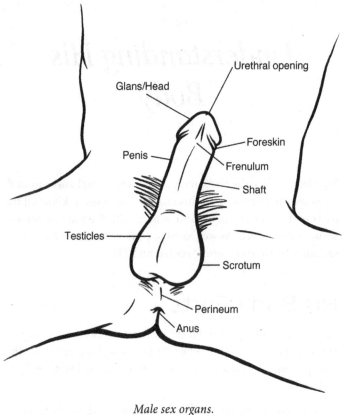

Male sex organs.

The Penis

The penis is a man's sexual and reproductive organ. Penises come in a variety of sizes, shapes, and colors. From long and skinny ones, short and chubby ones, curved ones, hairy or hairless ones, all penises are unique yet all function the same way. No matter what the penis looks like, a man should learn to love and accept it just the way it is, and his lover should learn to worship it. Always remember, it's not the size of it but what you can do with it that counts.

The two main parts of the penis are the shaft and the head (*glans*). The shaft contains the urethra, the tube that drains the bladder. The urethra stretches from the bladder to the urethral opening—where urine and semen exit, however not at the same time.

The word **glans** comes from the Latin word for "acorn."

The head of the penis, whether circumcised or not, is exposed when a penis is fully erect. This area has the largest concentration of nerve endings on the penis, and men enjoy extra oral stimulation around the head.

The Foreskin

All boys are born with a foreskin or a covering over the tip of the penis. If a penis is uncircumcised, this layer of skin will cover the head when the penis is soft (flaccid). Once it's erect, the foreskin will draw back to expose the head. The foreskin on a man is equivalent to the clitoral hood on a woman.

The Frenulum

Inside the foreskin is a layer of thin skin similar to the inner lips in women. Linking the foreskin to the penis is the *frenulum*, and this is where the foreskin is removed during a circumcision.

The frenulum is located just below the head on the underside of the penis, where the circumcision scar appears. If uncircumcised, the frenulum is in the same location, below the tip of his penis, where the inner skin of the foreskin's hood meets the outer skin of the penis. The frenulum is a hotbed of sensitive nerve endings.

The most sensitive area on a man's penis, his "sweet spot," is clinically referred to as the **frenulum.** This area calls for extra oral stimulation.

The Scrotum

The scrotum is located below the penis. Joined at the base of the penis, it is a puckered sac that hangs and houses the testicles. Most men do not have perfectly symmetrically hanging testicles, commonly referred to as balls. Usually one hangs a little lower than the other, and this is normal.

The scrotum protects the testicles from injury much like a helmet protects a motorcyclist's or a football player's head. The scrotum also works as a temperature control device. When it's cold, the muscles in the scrotum will contract, lifting the testicles protectively closer to his body. When the temperature heats up, it relaxes and lets them hang down. For the production of healthy sperm, the testicles need to be around 5 degrees below body temperature.

When a man gets fully aroused, just before ejaculation, the muscles in the scrotum will contract and his balls will rise, pulling them closer to the base of his penis. This is the point of no return.

The Testicles

Also known as the testes, the testicles are inside the scrotal sac behind the base of the penis. These globes of pleasure produce the sex hormone testosterone, as well as sperm. Regular ejaculation is healthy so older sperm can be released, leaving room for new sperm to be replenished.

Most men love having their testicles orally lavished, which should be done with great care since the testicles are fragile and highly sensitive.

> The testicles are about 4 or 5 degrees cooler than the rest of a man's body temperature, providing the perfect conditions for sperm production. Avoid sitting in hot tubs and wearing tight briefs if you're trying to conceive.

The Anus

The anus is below the scrotum at the opposite end of the perineum. As on a woman, a man's anus is surrounded by sensitive nerve endings making it a source of great pleasure for those daring enough to explore it, and to let it be explored. We will discuss oral stimulation techniques for the anus in detail in Chapter 9.

The H-Spot (Prostate)

Men have the equivalent of a woman's G-spot, I call it their H-spot for "hero spot." It's actually his prostate gland, which is located about 2 to 3 inches inside the anus (beneath the bladder). When stimulated, the prostate can provide orgasmic pleasure for some men, especially when it's combined with fellatio. We will cover techniques for arousal of the H-spot in Chapter 11.

A Healthy Penis, Scrotum, and Prostate

While a man's penis doesn't need to maintain a certain pH level to stay healthy, the way a woman's vagina does, a man does need to do his part to keep all of his equipment in good working order. Obviously, if you want your genitals to taste and smell their best, you should bathe just before your oral sex encounter. For uncircumcised men, it's important to pull back the foreskin of the penis and clean underneath it where dead skin can build up and create an unpleasant odor. Maintaining good hygiene is a man's best defense against fungal infections, such as jock itch. Checking himself regularly for any changes to his penis, testicles, prostate (noticed with urinary issues or impotence), and getting regular physical check-ups are essential for a man to ensure he stays healthy and in good sexual condition.

You Are What You Eat

If you intend to ejaculate in your lover's mouth—with her permission—you should be sure your sperm tastes as good as it can. So taste your own sperm. If you want a woman to taste you, then you should be prepared to taste yourself, too.

Lots of things affect the flavor of a man's semen, such as stress and other maladies. When you don't feel well, your body is not going to taste healthy. Also, semen of smokers taste more bitter than nonsmokers; and the semen of avid coffee drinkers, garlic and asparagus eaters, and even meat eaters tend to taste more acidic than others. To keep your semen smelling and tasting its best, drink lots of water and eat lots of fruit, especially pineapple and melons.

His Stages of Sexual Arousal

In Chapter 2, we introduced the study done by researchers Masters and Johnson of the sexual response cycle. Men's bodies actually respond differently sexually than women's, and the more you know about how both sexes respond, the more you'll be able to enhance your sexual experience for you both. The four stages of a man's sexual arousal cycle leading to orgasm are:

Stage #1: Excitement. Whether his sexual excitement is created by physical or mental stimulation, the result is the same. His blood flow is increased to his genitals, and the penis, perineum, and prostate begin to harden. His heart, pulse, and respiration rate raise, too.

Stage #2: Plateau. The head of his penis becomes engorged with blood and swells. For the uncircumcised man, the penis head pushes out of the hole in the foreskin. At the urethral opening, some men secrete more pre-ejaculatory fluid than others, which is commonly known as "pre-come." This fluid contains semen, so practice all the necessary safer sex precautions to protect yourself and your lover from STDs and pregnancy.

Stage #3: Orgasm. His blood pressure rises and muscle tension builds to a peak as he's about to reach his orgasm. The testicles rise up close to his penis while his prostate gland is filled with fluid, ready to burst. When his involuntary pelvic muscular contractions begin, there's no going back and the sperm shoots out of the urethral opening of his penis.

Stage #4: Resolution. This is when the body goes back to its normal pre-arousal state. Muscles relax, the penis becomes soft, and the testicles descend back to their usual place. Heart beat and breathing slows down, and lots of men feel so relaxed that they just want to go to sleep.

It's normal for men to feel sexually depleted after their orgasm. They need time (between 10 to 20 minutes) to regenerate their energy and their sperm. Some food and a beverage will help refuel the body after orgasm. We'll explore orgasms in more detail in Chapter 7.

The resolution cycle is different for a man because he needs to rest, whereas a woman can continue to have more orgasms if vaginal or clitoral stimulation continues.

Better He Be Safe Than Sorry

Many people are unclear on the risks associated with oral sex. While unprotected oral sex carries a lesser risk for the transmission of STDs than unprotected intercourse or anal penetration, there's still a risk of it for both the giver and the receiver of oral sex. Let's look at what supplies men can use to protect themselves, and their partners.

Male Condoms

Male condoms provide both oral sex partners protection from the transmission of STDs. Condoms are waterproof and elastic, and most are made out of latex or polyurethane. Lambskin or natural condoms should be avoided because they are not effective in the prevention of STDs.

Condoms today are high-tech wonders, featuring anatomically sophisticated shapes, innovative designs, and space age materials, not to mention a variety of colors, sizes, and flavors. There is a condom out there to suit any possible need, desire, or fetish imaginable.

Store condoms in a cool, dark place. Exposure to sunlight, heat, or humidity can break down latex, causing it to rupture or tear more easily. Unopened condoms are usable up to four years after the date of manufacture. Always check the date. If a condom breaks, try to figure out why the condom broke so you can prevent it from happening again.

Trojan, LifeStyles, Durex, and Trustex are all popular brands of condoms. The website www.condomania.com has a wide variety of pleasurable condoms and lubricants.

Lubricants

We all know "wetter is better," so use some lubricant with your safer sex supplies. It can be very confusing to know which lube, oil, or potion is best for your needs because there are so many to choose from. I suggest an odorless, tasteless, water-soluble lubricant with a lighter consistency and without Nonoxynol-9 spermicide (it's thought that it may actually increase the risk of STD transmission). Some of my favorite lubricants are: Wet Light, Astroglide, ForePlay Personal Gel, Aqua Lube, Sensua Organics, Probe Silky Light, System JO Lube, and Sex Butter.

Good Head Gel by Doc Johnson Enterprises is one of my favorite oral sex enhancements. It's for people who want to add some pizzazz to the flavor of their partner's genitals. It's available in mint, cinnamon, cherry, strawberry, and passion fruit flavors. It's worth buying for the "The History of Fellatio" article that comes inside the 4-ounce box.

4

Getting Ready to Go Down

Now that you have a better understanding about what and where everything is, let's set the mood for oral sex. In this chapter, you'll learn everything you need to know before you go down—there's more to it than soft lighting and sexy music. If you psyche yourself up for oral sex in different ways, it will greatly impact your sexual experience. How to do that is all in this chapter. You'll also learn how to make condoms an erotic part of your oral sex experience, as well as how to talk sexy and communicate what you want.

Setting the Mood

Just like getting ready to watch the Super Bowl game, preparation is the key to having an enjoyable and more memorable time. For instance, for the Super Bowl, you'd want to have a well-situated big-screen TV, some comfortable seats and pillows, the right temperature in the room, lots of food, and plenty to drink. Now let's use the same analogy for setting the mood for oral sex. The right atmosphere can turn any night into an evening your lover won't forget. A few small preparations to create a good atmosphere for oral sex will make all the difference.

Let's start with where you'll be having oral sex. Whether it's in bed, on the couch, on the floor, or some other exotic place, it's important that it's clean. Add a romantic ambience with dimmed lights and candles. Use however many candles you'd like, if they are scented ensure the scent is not overwhelming. Fresh flowers are a nice touch. Soft pillows are an inviting addition to lounge on. You can throw them on the bed, sofa, even on the floor. Music is definitely important. Have CDs or a music mix ready to play that's pleasing to you both. Ask your lover what kind of music gets him or her in the mood beforehand. Anything by Barry White, Sade, Andrea Bocelli, or Luther Vandross is a good bet.

Music is one of the things that people remember the most from receiving oral sex.

Even if you go out for dinner first, you might get hungry after oral sex, so have some fresh fruit or perhaps a decadent dessert on hand to enjoy afterwards. Don't forget to have handy something to wet your whistle—one of oral sex's necessities.

Your safer sex supplies should be close at hand including condoms, dental dams, latex gloves, finger cots, and lubricants. A box of tissues, baby wipes, or a clean hand towel at arm's reach will keep you from having to get up afterwards.

Getting Psyched Up

Psyching yourself up for anything prepares you mentally and emotionally, sometimes even physically. Whatever the challenge is, you will be more capable of dealing with it. For example, before running a marathon, you would want to increase your physical endurance through cardiovascular exercise, increase your strength with weight training, watch what you eat, get plenty of sleep, and visualize yourself winning the marathon. You have to expect to win, because if you prepare for success, you will get what you expect.

The fact that you've picked up this book means you've taken the right step in preparing yourself for going down. You have the desire to learn everything you can to be a good lover, and you've taken action to make it happen. Now you just have to believe you can give it, receive it, and enjoy it, and you will achieve all of it.

To help get you psyched up, it's helpful to understand what type of individual you are, as well as your partner, so you can approach oral sex with even greater understanding and overcome fears or anxieties about going down.

The Reluctant

In sex, it has been said that those who have the courage to communicate and experiment will find the greatest gratification. If you are reluctant to give or receive oral sex, ask yourself why before rejecting it completely. If your reluctance stems from sexual shame or guilt, these negative attitudes can be changed into positive ones as long as you have the desire to change them.

If you genuinely don't like oral sex, then read no farther, because I don't believe anyone should do anything they don't want to. If, however, you have had some prior unpleasant experiences sexually, don't punish yourself or your new lover by being reluctant to enjoy oral pleasure with someone who's now right for you. Disregard negative statements about the genitals being unclean, or advice of peers who have cautioned you that oral sex is taboo or sinful. Even though it's hard to shake these views as an adult, you have the ability to reprogram yourself. Start by admitting that your peers didn't know any better and realize that they probably said those things because that's what they were taught.

Create a relaxing atmosphere for yourself before you begin your voyage into oral sex. Meditate, relax in a bubble bath, get a therapeutic message, take a long walk, listen to music, or do whatever it takes to get yourself prepared for a satisfying sexual journey.

The Novice

As a novice, you may have little or no experience at oral sex, but you are receptive, not reluctant. It's important for you to choose the right partner, someone who is patient and worthy of your oral sex affections. Get to know this person as well as you can before you indulge in oral sex. To psyche yourself up, imagine you are watching a big screen of your oral sex adventures. Visualize what your partner is doing to you and what you are doing to him or her. Your partner is responding positively to everything you do. Both of you are having a great time. Use all your senses to feel the experience of giving and receiving oral sex; touch your body lovingly, smell your lover's natural scent, look at his or her body erotically, taste your lover's genitals, and hear your lover groaning with pleasure. You will discover that the mind is the most erotic organ we have.

The Amateur

This is someone who has already experimented and had good, mediocre, or not-so-good encounters. Whatever you experienced in the past, ask yourself what you learned. If it wasn't great, ask yourself what would have made it better. Every person is unique, so don't make the mistake of comparing your past partners with your present one, especially out loud. Don't assume your new lover will be aroused in exactly the same way as your past lover, or even that you will have the same sexual experience as you had before. If you did something that drove your last lover wild in bed, there's no guarantee that it will have the same effect on your new lover. Enjoy the newness of your lover by exploring all his or her erogenous zones with your tongue. Don't be shy to let your lover know that you want to give the best oral sex he or she has ever had.

The Experienced

The experienced person enjoys the art of oral sex and doesn't need to prepare psychologically in the same way as the other three do. However, it's important to maintain curiosity whether you're with your lover for the first time or the hundredth time.

Always ask questions like, "What's your favorite oral sex position?" and don't be afraid to ask for constructive criticism and feedback. As an experienced oral lover, you must be sure you don't become too predictable, so maintain enthusiasm and be willing to try new things. Even if your partner isn't responsive to giving you feedback, be sure you communicate your needs openly and honestly. Chances are your partner will catch on.

What to Say in the Beginning

So how do you bring up the subject of oral sex? You can't just blurt out, "I want to get some head," unless you never want to see that date again. Some people consider oral sex more intimate than intercourse, while others view it just as foreplay. It's up to you to find out how your partner feels about giving and getting oral sex. The best way to start an intimate discussion like this is to talk about your thoughts on the subject. If you think oral sex is a prelude to intercourse, you can say, "One of the sexiest things about making love for me is giving and getting oral sex before we make love. What do you think?" This is an open-ended question, so your lover has to give you a substantial answer. Whatever his or her answer, be sure you acknowledge it and don't be judgmental.

For example, a guy may respond by saying, "When I'm getting oral sex, I often get carried away and reach an orgasm before I want to." He may be feeling inadequate as a lover and blaming himself for having *premature ejaculation*. You can help him by letting him know that it's okay. Say, "We'll go slowly and you can tap me on the shoulder when you think you're going to come and then I'll get on top of you, rub my clit against your shaft, so we can climax together at the same time." He'll be reassured that you're getting your needs met and that he's okay just the way he is. If your response had been unkind or insensitive, it could make his premature ejaculation even worse.

Premature ejaculation is when a man is not in control over the timing of his ejaculation and believes that it occurs too soon.

A woman might say, "Getting oral sex is the only sure way I know how to climax," in which case the guy can reply, "That's great. I'll go down on you first, and then you can do me." Another sure way to help build a woman's confidence is to say something like, "You look so delicious, I can hardly wait to taste you."

Making Condoms Sexy

Guys can make any number of excuses for not wanting to wear a condom, "It's unromantic," "It falls off," and my favorite, "If she really likes me, she won't make me use one." The truth is, condoms provide safety to both partners against STDs, so if you're not in a monogamous relationship, they are an important part of your sexual experience, however they don't have to spoil all the fun. Make condoms *part* of the fun by learning to put a condom on your partner's penis with your mouth. This can be an erotic experience in itself.

First it's a good idea to get some flavored condoms. Trustex has a large variety of scented and flavored condoms. Pick your favorite flavor from banana, strawberry, orange, vanilla, cherry, or spearmint. Next, follow these steps to make putting it on an experience he won't want to forget:

1. Get his penis erect.

2. Put a drop of lubricant on the head of his penis.

3. Carefully remove the condom from the package.

4. Place the condom inside your mouth with the receptacle end lightly resting on top of your tongue. Leave some room at the end for the semen.

5. Be sure the condom is inverted in your mouth so it will go on correctly when placed on his penis.

6. Push the condom onto the head of his penis using your lips, not your teeth.

7. Wrap your lips around the head of his penis and use a little suction on the end of the receptacle of the condom to insure enough room for semen.

You may want to practice putting a condom on a cucumber, banana, or plastic dildo before you attempt it on your lover's penis. Practice makes perfect, so have fun making safer sex enjoyable for both of you.

Sexy Talk

Aural sex is to the ears what a mirror is to the eyes, it's intimate and erotic talk. Telling your lover what you like or dislike, or asking him or her what stimulation they enjoy doesn't have to be nerve-racking or embarrassing if you haven't done it before. It enables you to direct your lover to pleasure you exactly the way you want. Remember, he or she can't read your mind.

There's nothing wrong with telling your lover how you like or dislike to receive oral sex. If you don't like to have your testicles licked or sucked, say so up front, then she won't go there. If the only way you can reach an orgasm is by having your clitoris softly licked, then admit it before he gets started.

5

Pleasuring Her

In this chapter, we'll explore oral sex foreplay and essential moves for performing oral sex on a woman. You will also be introduced to different ways to stimulate her with your tongue. Then we move on to an explanation of some introductory positions for oral sex as well as what you can do with your hands.

Working Your Way Down

While you may want to get right to the main event, keep in mind that a lot of women want foreplay before oral sex. It can help them relax and get in the mood for it. That isn't to say that some women don't want you to go right for the gold every time. However, to enhance your chances of success, it's best if you start out slow, giving her a chance to get ready. Start by kissing her lips, her neck, her breasts—get her really hot and turned on while you're heading south. The anticipation you create as you work your way down her body is sure to tease and arouse her even more.

Once you get past her belly and arrive at her vagina, start things off with a sexy compliment. "You have the sexiest vagina." (See

Chapter 1 for a discussion on what you can call her vagina.) We all like to hear how attractive someone finds us, and that's not just from the waist up. Also, when you compliment her, you're helping her relax, which not only makes her feel better, it makes your job easier. A woman who feels confident and trusting is much easier to arouse than one who is feeling uptight and insecure.

Scent of a Woman

What do you do when you arrive at her vagina and something isn't quite right? It's that dreaded four-letter word—odor. First of all, let me say this: The myth of the smelly vagina is just that—a myth. All our body parts have the potential to be clean or dirty, malodorous or odor-free. The vagina is no exception. Many men find the scent of their lover's vagina quite sexy. On the other hand, if you do go down on a woman who is emitting a strong scent, keep in mind this may be a sign that she has an STD or an infection. If that's the case, take this as a warning sign, and instead of using your mouth, consider using your hands to stimulate her vagina.

Assuming all things are healthy, and you run into the problem of odor, you may want to suggest to your lover that you take a shower together. Invite her to shower or take a bubble bath with you. Tell her you want to feel intimate with her before being sexual. Make it into a rewarding experience, not a punishment.

If you prefer a quick fix, all the major lubricant companies now manufacture flavored lubes in a variety of flavors. You're sure to find one you like. Apply a small amount to her clitoris, and you're in business. Some people prefer the odor and taste of flavored lubes to the natural smell and flavor of their partner. Flavored lube may also decrease your partner's inhibitions about oral sex because she won't be worried about odors.

What to Do When You Get There

When it comes to women, a slow seductive hand can rarely go wrong. Start by massaging her vaginal lips, gently running your finger along the seam where her lips come together. It may take a few minutes for you to get her really turned on and get her wet, so don't get discouraged. If you do this right, you'll probably inspire her to press herself into your hand, your wrist, your arm. This is a good thing. Once she's this turned on, you know she's ready for you to move in with your mouth and tongue.

Her Vulva

Start kissing her vulva, or mons (the soft area above her vagina that is covered with pubic hair or shaved of hair), working your way down from the top. The goal is not to miss a single place. If it helps, imagine you're kissing her face. Place delicate kisses where each cheek would be, where her eyelids would be, her forehead, her temples, her nose, her jaw, and her mouth. Continue until you've kissed the equivalent of her entire face. You may even want to give her a nibble here and there. Be sure not to bite too hard at first. If she asks for more pressure, don't be shy. Your job is to abide by her wishes.

Now it's time to put that tongue to use. Run the flat of your tongue across her mons from bottom to top. Be sure you address both sides. You want to be sure she feels stimulated all over. After a couple minutes of kissing and licking, you can feel confident in moving on to the next step.

Her Vaginal Lips

Trace the point of your tongue along the crease where her vaginal lips come together. Take one of her outer lips in your mouth and gently tug on it with your lips. Begin sucking, softly at first, building with her degree of excitement. You may even want to gently nibble on them. Alternately drag your teeth across her outer lips then suck. Nibble (gently) then lick. The variation in pressure and sensation will serve as a pleasant tease.

It's important to note here that some women absolutely lose their minds when you suck on their vaginal lips and some wonder why you're even wasting your time. So don't be put off if she doesn't respond. However, if she's one of those women who can't get enough, stick with it. She'd be more than happy for you to lick, nibble, and suck for a few minutes. Don't forget to repeat all that attention on the opposite side as well.

Working your way from outside in, you now find yourself at her inner vaginal lips. Hold her outer lips open with each hand as you press your mouth into her inner lips. Trace each side with the tip of your tongue, stimulating her with circular movements. Lick her from bottom to top with the flat of your tongue. Make your tongue dance around. Let your excitement add to and inspire her excitement.

The inner vaginal lips are more sensitive than the vulva or the outer vaginal lips. Although each woman has her own preferences, biting here may prove rather painful for most. So you may not want to experiment with nibbling and love bites in this sensitive area unless she specifically asks you.

As she presses herself against you, slip your tongue inside her vagina, working your way up toward her clitoris.

Exploring Her Clitoris

There are countless ways to stimulate a woman's clitoris. The important thing to remember is that she's in charge. Let her tell you whether she'd like it fast or slow, harder or softer, to the right or the left, up or down, or whatever combination she likes. If she's a little hesitant to instruct you, ask her. Asking, "Baby, tell me what turns you on," is a turn-on in itself. Now, having said all that, there are some techniques you can use to stimulate her clitoris and give her an experience she won't soon forget.

Licking

The most basic cunnilingus technique is licking. A lot of people tend to use repetitive, quick, short strokes to the clitoris. There is nothing wrong with this technique, but there are other options as well. Use your entire tongue, dragging it across her clitoris from the base all the way to the point. Move your tongue from side to side like windshield wipers. Try circular motions as well, both around her clitoris and on it. Turn your head to the side, alternating again between licking in quick, short strokes and slowly dragging your tongue across her clit from base to point. Don't be afraid to come at her from a different angle!

Sucking

A client of mine once told me a story about going down on a woman and having the feeling that he was doing nothing for her. Exasperated, he finally sat up and declared, "I suck!" "No, you don't," the woman replied. Actually, she, as many women do, liked the feeling of having her clitoris sucked. If this seems odd, just think of her clitoris like a nipple, which is very receptive to being sucked. Simply wrap your lips around her clitoris and start sucking. The results are nearly immediate. She'll either swoon with delight or possibly flinch in pain. Don't let a flinch throw you completely off. She may just prefer you to suck more lightly as opposed to not at all. Start off sucking lightly, and let her tell you how far to go with it.

When a woman is close to reaching her orgasm, you need to keep your tongue and rhythm at the same pace and in the same place. Don't change a thing until she stops you.

Moaning

Mmmmmm—it's not just a sound, it's a sensation. A woman wants to hear when you're between her thighs giving her oral sex that you're enjoying it. Sure, there are a variety of ways you can let her know this, but here's why mmmm, mmmm is at the top of my list: Not only does it let her know you're enjoying the way she tastes, smells, and feels, but she will also be able to feel the vibration of the mmmm, mmmm sound you make, which is even more arousing. With two sources of pleasure, it's twice as much fun for her.

Flipping Your Tongue

If you already know how to flip your tongue upside down, from the left and the right, you can use this technique right away. If you don't or need to learn it again, start by practicing in front of a mirror. You want to be able to turn your tongue upside down, preferably from both sides. When you're ready for the real deal, start by lining up the point of your tongue with her clitoris. As you spin your tongue, you will be essentially tracing the outside of her clitoris in alternating directions. Once you get the hang of it, throw in a lick or a suck between rotations. This little maneuver is sure to please her.

If flipping your tongue over is something you can't even visualize, let alone master, there are alternatives. Circle her clit with the tip of your tongue. Then change directions, and circle the other way.

Hand and Finger Work

Whether you're kissing her mons or licking her clitoris, your hands and fingers can be busy, too. Here are a few suggestions for how you can use them to increase her pleasure.

Double Stimulation

Try licking her perineum (the area of skin between her anus and her vagina) while rubbing her clitoris with your thumb. It may be easiest for her to bend one leg and for you to approach her from behind. Rest your head on her thigh as you run your tongue along her perineum, licking in long broad strokes. With the flat part of your tongue, lick her from the anus to the vaginal opening. Then, with the point of your tongue, trace zigzags across her perineum, like a skier doing the slalom. At the same time, rub her clitoris with your thumb. The combination of these two stimuli will send her through the roof. For an added twist, try the reverse. Lick and suck her clitoris while rubbing her perineum. This, too, is truly a winning combination.

Massage

While licking or sucking her, you can massage her lower back in a gentle circular motion. Work your way down, massaging, rubbing, and holding her behind. It's amazing how much more aroused a woman can get from being rubbed, held, or caressed in just the right place. It's your job to find out which of those places work best for the woman you're with. It may be her stomach, her hips, her legs, who knows. Enjoy exploring them all to find out.

Going Inside

If you've been massaging and licking for a while now, she'll probably be begging you to insert one or two fingers into her vagina. Be sure your hands and fingers are clean first, then, go for it. Insert your middle finger in slow motion first, and then if she's very wet, insert your forefinger, too. This is how you can stimulate her G-spot, which we'll cover in more detail in Chapter 10.

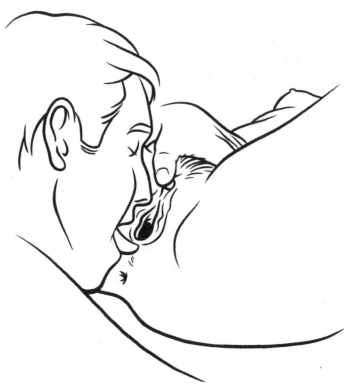

Double stimulation.

A Variety of Positions

When it comes to sex, we all have our personal favorite positions—
along with our very own favorite variations. Oral sex should be
no different. Here are some sexy oral sex positions for you to try,
hopefully you'll find new levels of pleasure with one or more of
them.

Lazy Susan. This is the basic oral sex position, with her on her
back and you on your stomach between her legs. This position
enables her to fully relax.

Hanging Hannah. This position is similar to Lazy Susan except
she hangs her legs over the side of the bed, and you kneel
between them. At this angle, you have greater access to more of
her vagina.

Shoulder stance. This is Lazy Susan with a twist. She lies on
her back. You kneel between her legs, and she raises her hips to
you. You should help her hold herself up. If you're feeling strong,
she may even throw her legs over your shoulders while you sup-
port her lower back. This isn't the easiest position to achieve, but
it's fun for a little variety. And again, the change in the angle of
your approach may stimulate her in unique ways.

Standing. This one's exactly as it sounds. She stands, you kneel.
Be kind and give her something to lean on—a wall or a piece
of furniture should do. If you're any good at what you do, she'll
need it!

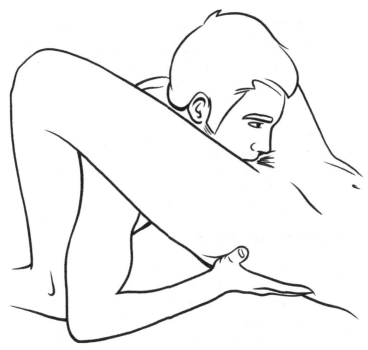

Shoulder stance.

Know When to Say When

If you've been down there a while, and bursting volcanoes don't seem to be just over the horizon, that's okay. It's important to remember you can't hit it out of the park every time you step up to the plate. Ask her if there's another way you can please her. Or, ask her if she'd like to please herself so you can watch.

Some women love kissing after you've gone down on them, others think it's gross. If you're not sure, start by kissing her breasts and working your way up to her neck, ears, and then around to her mouth. If she turns her head away or has a negative reaction, you'll know to quit. Who knows? Maybe she'll pull you in and want more.

It's no one's fault if she doesn't reach an orgasm. Oral sex can be great even if it doesn't end with an orgasm. The journey is to be enjoyed as much as the destination.

Watching Her

Most men love to look at women's bodies, and that includes their genitals. Why do you think so many *Playboy, Penthouse,* and *Hustler* magazines sell each month? It's not for the articles. If you want her to pleasure herself in front of you, you have to help make her feel secure about the way she looks. Start by complimenting her face and body, then let her know how much she turns you on. Ask her to tease you by rubbing herself over her underwear first. If she's too uncomfortable to do that, she's probably not going to masturbate for you, so it's best not to push it.

If she agrees, reward her with more compliments as she caresses herself, then ask her to slide her panties to one side so you can see more. It's a good idea for you to pleasure yourself at the same time so she can watch your erection grow. Mutual masturbation is highly erotic and educational because you can watch each other stroke yourselves, and then learn how and where your lover wants to be touched.

Getting Your Turn

If you want to ensure you get your turn in the oral pleasure spectrum, here's how you can entice her to go down on you:

Look your best. Keep your body clean and well groomed. Trim your pubic hair; better yet, shave your testicles. You know you like it when she is groomed and sweet-smelling for you. Give her the same courtesy.

Go down on her first. This is an excellent way to break the ice. You may even be able to slip into 69 in the process. Or you may make her feel so fantastic she'll be begging to return the favor.

Find what she likes. Some women just aren't into oral sex, as much as you. So offering to go down on her to inspire her to go down on you just isn't going to cut it. So you're just going to have to use a different currency. Figure out what she likes. It may be massages, going for picnics, dancing—whatever. It's your job to find out what pleases her so she'll want to please you.

{ Have fun! }

6

Pleasuring Him

This chapter teaches you how to "go down" and orally love your man. We'll also explore why wetter is better, all about sucking, and how hand signals can communicate your oral needs.

Getting Down to Business

Men typically don't want you to take the long way around and they don't want to play games when it comes to sex. Simply stated, men want to know that they are going to get some head. So feel free to get right down to business, literally.

To get into a basic position, he should lie on his back while you lie on your stomach between his legs. Relax and get comfortable, because you want this to be enjoyable for you, too.

Take his penis in your hand and hold it with confidence. Look at it lovingly and sensually. Don't be afraid of it. Your lover's penis is his pride and joy, and it's your job to validate it, when it's hard or soft, by kissing it, stroking it, licking it, and sucking it to keep it happy. If his hygiene isn't up to par, suggest taking a shower or bath together. If he already looks appetizing, give him a verbal compliment right away like, "You look so good. I can hardly wait to go down on you." Every man wants to hear that.

> If you are not in a monogamous relationship, practice safe sex and use a condom, even for oral sex. Chapters 2 and 3 include information on safer sex practices and devices.

If your lover is comfortable with letting you see his penis when it's not aroused, you don't need to wait until he has an erection before taking him into your mouth. He certainly won't stop you. While his penis is still soft, you can wrap your lips around it and take it into your mouth so you can get used to it before it grows to its full potential.

Now let's explore how to stimulate all the different areas of his genitals.

Giving a Blow Job

Start by making sure you have plenty of saliva in your mouth (a dry blow job is as bad as no blow job). Drink some water if you need to. Cover your teeth by wrapping your lips around them, then push your mouth down on your lover's penis, sucking (in slow motion) with your lips tightly closed (like sucking hard on a thick milkshake to get the drink through the straw). Guys like to feel the sensation of a wet, warm, tight mouth sucking his penis.

To go to the next level, open your mouth wide, relax your throat and move your mouth as far down over his penis shaft as you can, even if this is only for a few strokes, it will let him know you are willing to try *deep-throating*. Don't use your hands yet. Hands can come into play, and we'll get into that later on in this chapter as well.

To **deep-throat** someone is a form of oral sex in which the penis is voluntarily taken deeply down into the recipient's throat.

While his penis is in your mouth, don't forget to breathe. Inhale through your nose every time you suck his penis into your mouth and then exhale through your nose as you lift your chin and release the penis. Also don't forget to swallow your own saliva frequently because it creates a distinct tugging sensation on his penis and adds more pressure around it. If his penis makes you feel like you are choking or gagging, move his penis to the side of your mouth into the hollow of your cheeks and take some deep breaths. Some men are flattered when a woman gags on their penis because it makes him feel like he is well endowed.

A quick exercise to relax your jaw is to thrust your jaw forward, then down, then back, then to original position. You may want to do these when you're taking a break from the action. It's quick, easy, and will get you back into the oral swing of things.

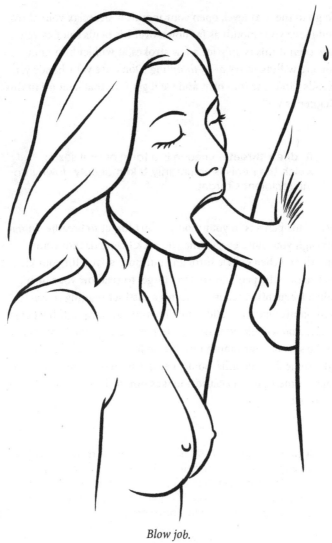

Blow job.

Continue lavishing your man's penis with long, deep, sucking motions. Let him know you're enjoying it, too, by maintaining sexy eye contact and moaning pleasurably. If you want to change positions, ask him to hang his legs over the side of the bed, and you kneel between them with a pillow under your knees for comfort.

The urethral opening, located on top of the penis head, is a very sensitive area. Run the tip of your tongue over it from side to side like a windshield wiper. Don't overdo it though, and don't try to wiggle your tongue inside the urethral opening because that's not sexy.

The Penis Head

The head of the penis (glans) is one of the most sensitive areas on a man, with many concentrated nerve endings.

Hold his penis at the base with your dominant hand and circle your tongue all the way around the head, clockwise then counterclockwise. Think of the head as a scoop of your favorite ice cream on top of a cone. You don't want to miss a drop of that tasty ice cream, so you greedily taste the top, lap up the sides, and lick all around his yummy penis.

The Frenulum

The frenulum is the most sensitive spot on the penis, so pay special attention to its location. Look on the underside of the head where the inner skin of the foreskin's hood meets in a heart shape. This is also where the circumcision scar appears (if uncircumcised, the frenulum is in the same place).

Begin by licking his frenulum from side to side with quick, darting flicks of your tongue. Then make an "O" with your lips around the frenulum and use your mouth to create some light suction on that area. Imagine you are sucking a clam out of its shell. Feel free to making sucking noises, because men love sexy sound effects.

The Raphe

The raphe is the penis seam, and it runs all the way from the head of the penis to the scrotum. It's even easy to find in the dark because you can feel the ridge of the seam with your fingers and your tongue. The raphe gives you an opportunity to lick his penis just like you would a lollipop, with long slurps. Start at the base of his penis, stick your tongue out as far as possible, and following the raphe, lick your way to the top of his penis. You can do this a few times to add some variety to your experience.

The Scrotum and Testicles

His scrotum (or sac) and testicles (or balls) are an important part of his sexual package, so don't ignore them. Get familiar with them by caressing and gently massaging these balls of pleasure.

Handle his testicles as if they are a precious artifact made of china. You want to admire them and hold them, but you don't want to damage them.

He can stand while you kneel in front of him or you can lie down on your back while he straddles you. The latter position is particularly good for access to his balls. You can kiss, lick, and suck on his scrotum by pulling it away from the testicles, which are inside the sac. Imagine you are sucking on your lover's bottom lip with your mouth and imitate that same technique on his scrotum. *But absolutely do not use your teeth.*

This can be highly erotic for him, and he may request this oral method over and over again. It's easy to do because there's no gagging effect, and to make it even more erotic for him, ask him to masturbate while you suck on his scrotum.

The testicles are delicate like fresh farm eggs, so approach them cautiously yet sensually. Begin licking one ball at a time with the flat of your tongue in circular motions all around it, letting your head follow suit (this is also a good neck exercise). Then give the other testicle equal attention until they are both sopping wet from your saliva. Next open your mouth wide and cup your lips gently around one of his balls while using the tip of your tongue to lick it in a circular action. Do the same to the other one and give them equal time. For the icing on the cake, use one of your hands to carefully push his testicles together and try to place them both in your mouth. You'll find even more testicle-sucking techniques in Chapter 11.

The Perineum

The perineum is located behind his penis (the stretch of skin between the anus and the scrotum), so it may be easier for you to access from behind. It is a totally erotic area for him.

Ask him to lie on his stomach with his legs spread apart, then slide in between his legs and run your tongue along his perineum. Start by using the top flat part of your tongue in long broad strokes to lick him from the anus to the scrotum and then use the lower flat part of your tongue to lick from the scrotum to the anus. Next, with the point of your tongue, trace zigzags across his perineum as if you were a professional skier on a mountain.

Oral Combinations

Stimulating more than one area simultaneously is an amazing experience for him. Learning some techniques to do it will automatically make you an oral sex guru. Here are ways you can pleasure your man in more than one area at once.

Strum His Violin

Slide your prominent hand beneath his testicles, cup them together, and gently caress them with your fingers (be careful with your nails). Then take his penis in the other hand, and hold it firmly while you flick your pointed tongue back and forth over his frenulum. Imagine you are a musician strumming a violin with your tongue to make beautiful music. Your man's moans and groans will confirm that you are playing it correctly.

Suck and Brush

The best position for this technique is the 69 position with you on top. Make a tight seal around the head of his penis with your mouth and suck as you draw your head back, releasing his penis. While you continue to suck your man's penis, brush your fingernails lightly against his perineum as if you were a cat clawing your way up a tree. Gently brush both sides of your fingernails lightly from one end of his sexual landing strip to the other.

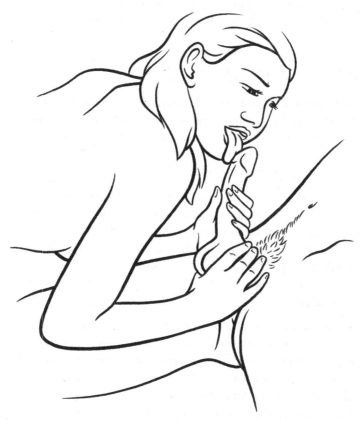

Strum his violin.

Bead It

Wrap a string of beads or pearls around his scrotum, and tug them gently while sucking the head. After a few minutes, let the beads dangle around his balls while you insert your index finger into your mouth and circle the head of his penis with it while you continue to suck on it. This stimulation makes a man feel like he's getting a blow job from two different people.

Why Wetter Is Better

If you want to enjoy giving oral sex, then you have to get used to the fact that it's going to be wet and sometimes sticky or messy. A man's penis does not have as much natural lubrication as a woman's vagina. Even with the pre-ejaculation fluid, it's not enough to masturbate him with.

The sexiest lubricant is your saliva, but don't just spit all over his penis. Drink some water if you feel dehydrated, fill your mouth with plenty of saliva, then let it drip over and down his penis as you take him into your mouth. You can rub it in with your hands if you are planning to masturbate him. No man wants a dry hand job. A man loves the feeling of warm, sloppy juices all over his penis.

Drink some hot liquid prior to giving him oral sex so you don't "run dry" and lack enough lubrication to give him maximum enjoyment. He'll love the hot, steamy feeling around his penis. You can also gargle with mouthwash or suck on a mint prior to going down on him for a tingly fresh feeling you'll both enjoy. If things are getting too hot, suck on crushed ice while you give him oral sex. It will keep you from getting dry mouth and give him a frosty thrill.

Using Your Hands

One of the best things about using your hands is that you can use them as an extension of your mouth. They're especially handy if you don't want to or can't deep-throat him. There's no doubt you will want to use your hands to steady his penis while you worship it orally. Hand contact also enables you to sensually caress other parts of his body such as his nipples and testicles while you're down there.

Your hands can play with his testicles as well as guide his penis in any direction you want and keep it from going too deep. Your hands can even mimic your mouth's actions if your jawbone gets too tired. But you'll need to use plenty of lubricant on your hands so he feels the warm moisture around his penis.

If you want to give your guy a great hand job, ask him to masturbate with you watching so you can see how he likes it. Put your hand over his hand and try to duplicate his grip and the amount of pressure he uses. You can start a hand job by stroking his penis up and then down, but remember that men prefer a smoother, rapid motion without stopping between strokes. The phrase "jerking off" is confusing because men don't really like a jerking motion at all.

When he ejaculates, don't stop masturbating him immediately unless he asks you to. Most guys appreciate a few extra strokes as they are reaching their climax. Don't be shy to ask him to show you what turns him on. He'll be impressed that you care and want to learn.

There is a playful side to using your hands, too. Let your fingers dance around his genitals as you run them around his testicles and up and down his shaft. Wet your fingers with your saliva, then stroke the outside of his anus and tickle his perineum. Pump him up by squeezing his penis in the palm of your hand. And last but not least, give him a hand job with a twisting motion from the base to the tip, as if you were twisting half of an orange on a juicer. Guys tell me that this method of stimulation is the cat's meow.

Sex Signals

Signals can be very useful, particularly when your mouth is full and you can't talk. Agree on various sex signals with your partner before you go down or before you do something you're initially uncomfortable with. Examples of sex signals are him letting you know that he's about to climax by patting you on the shoulder so you have time to move your mouth if you don't want to swallow. You can tap each other on the belly or back gently or more energetically as a signal to go slower or faster. Point your right forefinger to the right when you want your lover to move slightly to the right and move your left forefinger to the left when you want your lover to move slightly to the left. Stick your thumb up in the "OK" sign to communicate "don't move," and clap your hands in a gentle applause to signify, "that it feels great."

Where He Comes

Men love to climax inside their lover's mouth. But if you don't want to swallow or don't enjoy the taste of semen, here's a little trick that could save the moment. As soon as you get the sign that he's about to climax, whether he's tapping you on the shoulder or you feel his testicles rising, flip your tongue on top of his penis as opposed to keeping it under his penis. This will prevent his semen from spurting on to the side of your tongue where the majority of your taste buds are located. Keep your lips tightly wrapped around the head of his penis as you change the position of your tongue, and he'll never notice the difference. An alternative is to let him come in your mouth and then discreetly spit his semen into a towel close by.

Some men like to watch their semen squirt out, so they prefer to climax on a woman's face, breasts, tummy, or pubic mound. If you don't want to experience his ejaculation on you, then slide your mouth to his frenulum as he is climaxing so his semen will shoot toward his own stomach. If he's using a condom, the semen will be contained inside it.

Getting Your Turn

It's up to you to encourage your lover to go down south. Some go willingly, while others are clueless or apprehensive. Here are some things to try when you're ready to get your turn.

Give a gentle nudge. When the guy is kissing your breasts or stomach, you should do the same thing that he often does: gently guide his head toward your vagina by pushing him there. He'll get the point.

Make some noise. Moan like crazy, or scream if you want to. Who cares what the neighbors think. Let him know it's pleasurable as he gets closer, from breasts, to stomach, and so on. No guy will stop if he hears his efforts recognized.

Talk dirty. "Eat me," "Lick me harder," "Flick your tongue softly on my clit," "Suck my lips as hard as you can and tickle my clit," "Finger my G-spot and suck my clit softly." Take the guesswork out of it and tell your lover what feels good.

Suggest a 69. Better still, just get on top of him in the 69 position and start giving him a blow job while you sit on his face. He's probably not going to have a problem reciprocating.

Watch porn. Show him how much you can get off when a woman is being eaten properly. Porn will also let him see how it's done.

However, some guys simply aren't into giving oral sex. For guys who don't like it, you can try teasing him with kisses and tastes of a flavored lubricant or gel and then put it on your clit and direct him there. It's the idea of objectionable taste that freaks some guys out about oral sex. Or it may be a matter of social upbringing and confidence for others that keep them from doing it. Whatever the reason, with open communication and patience, you can bring him around to it, one lick at a time.

Have fun!

7

Exploring Orgasms

Obviously, having an amazing orgasm, or orgasms, is where we all want to end up. In this chapter, we'll explore how to achieve mind-blowing orgasms and how to create your orgasm pleasure scale. You'll discover the benefits of orgasms and understand what can prevent you from reaching one.

There are actually lots of different types of orgasms to choose from, and we'll discuss five you won't want to miss out on. We'll also explore the juicy subject of sex fluids like semen, saliva, vaginal fluids, and female ejaculation and how sexy they can be.

What Is an Orgasm?

Orgasm is wired to our brain before it travels between our legs. It's a combination of emotional and most often, physical events that signal the brain to activate the body to experience involuntary physical responses, including:

- Increased breathing, additional blood flow to the genitals, and rapid heart rate

- Muscular contraction around the vagina, prostate, and anus

- The penis becoming erect and the vagina moist

- Men usually ejaculating as well as some women

Refer to the section on the male and female sexual arousal cycles in Chapters 2 and 3 for more details on how an orgasm affects the male and female body.

So why are we seeking that euphoric, mind-blowing, earth-shattering, energy-melting experience of the orgasm, over and over again? Because we can't help it. It is our second basic human instinct after self-preservation (survival).

We also seek to lose that part of ourselves that connects us to the everyday and mundane. For a brief moment, we can lose the pain and hassle of being human and become one with the universe while we float on air like gods.

Your Orgasm Pleasure Scale

Imagine you have a personal pleasure scale ranging from numbers 1 to 10, with 1 being the minimum amount of arousal you can feel and 10 being the point of no return—orgasm. Now let's compare your pleasure scale to the Empire State Building, which has 102 floors. Picture the tenth floor as your number 1 on your pleasure scale and the 102nd floor as your number 10. There's a long way to go before you get to the reward of standing on the balcony and looking out at the beautiful view. Of course, some people will take the elevator and miss out on the experience of climbing 102 floors, while others will enjoy the journey and create anticipation of their arrival.

It's a good idea for everyone to recognize their levels of arousal so they become familiar with how their body functions, discovering what turns them on the most. For example, getting a massage may only take you to a level 2 on your pleasure scale, whereas being kissed may take you to a level 4. Then masturbating may take you to a level 5, but mutual masturbation takes you to a level 6. Giving oral sex could take you to a level 7, and receiving oral sex may take you all the way to level 10. You are in control of your own pleasure scale, and you can learn a lot by watching your lover go up and down on his or her pleasure scale, too.

Take the time to create your personal pleasure scale and help your partner do the same. This is a wonderful exercise that will enhance your relationship in the communication, intimacy, and sexual departments. Sexual knowledge results in sexual satisfaction.

Types of Orgasms

There are many different kinds of orgasm you can experience from stimulation of different parts of your body. Each one will create different kinds of feelings, ranging from quick, short, localized, deep, concentrated, to full-body orgasms. Oral sex gives you the perfect opportunity to experiment with as many different kinds of orgasm as you can.

If you have never experienced an orgasm, you may be suffering from gynecological, urological, hormonal, or neurological disorders, so check with your medical practitioner first. If everything is in good working condition, then it's possible you have a psychological block such as a traumatic past sexual experience, resentment toward your partner, guilt, fears, inhibitions, or other negative feelings. With the help of a professional sexologist, sex counselor, or therapist, you can overcome your blocks and open the door to the world of orgasms.

A UniGasm, Nipple Style

A UniGasm is an orgasm resulting from stimulation directed to one primary erogenous zone such as the penis, testicles, clitoris, G-spot, anus, or nipples.

In this example, let's focus on how nipple stimulation (for men and women) can produce an orgasm. While it's not as common as some of the other erogenous zones, it's just as enjoyable.

For women, having their breasts caressed and nipples sucked releases oxytocin, the chemical that makes them feel like they are in love.

Many men enjoy stimulating a woman's nipples during foreplay but rarely think of them as having orgasmic potential, but they certainly do. To give memorable oral sex on her breasts and nipples, understand that the size of her breasts have nothing to do with their sensitivity, they are sensitive regardless of size.

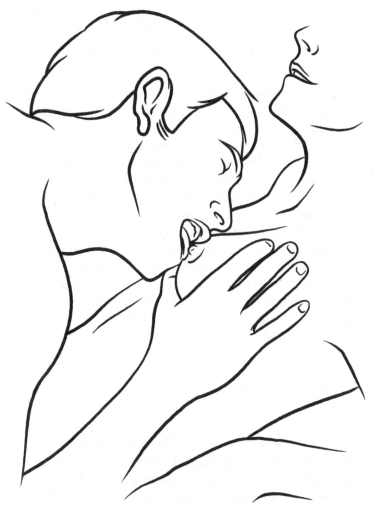

Female nipple stimulation.

As a woman, if you are not turned on by having your breasts or nipples played with then guide your partner to another erogenous zone that does turn you on.

Begin by caressing and licking both of her breasts, not just her nipples. Alternate each one as you use the flat of your tongue in lapping motions all around her breasts, covering every centimeter. Follow your tongue with light fingertip caresses, saving her nipples until last. When both breasts are suitably wet from your tongue, cup your hand over one breast at a time so the tip of her nipple rests in between your thumb and your index finger. Squeeze your fingers together so you raise her nipple slightly and then begin licking it with the tip of your tongue in circular motions. After about a dozen or so licks, pucker your lips around the nipple and suck gently, but firmly, letting your head bob up and down simultaneously. Don't forget to give equal attention to both breasts and nipples. When she is climaxing, do not stop or change what you are doing. Let her push you away when she is ready.

To enhance oral nipple sensation, try putting an ice cube in your mouth while lavishing them orally.

For male nipple stimulation, the directions are pretty much the same, except men are more interested in having immediate nipple contact with deeper vacuum-sucking motions from the woman, not so much teasing around the nipple area. Some men even enjoy having their nipples nibbled on. So ladies, it's up to you to find out how much pain or pleasure your man wants on his nipples. Some men have one nipple that is more sensitive than the other. While you suck on one, you can pinch the other one and then ask him which one feels most erotic. You could be the first one to introduce him to a UniGasm through his nipples.

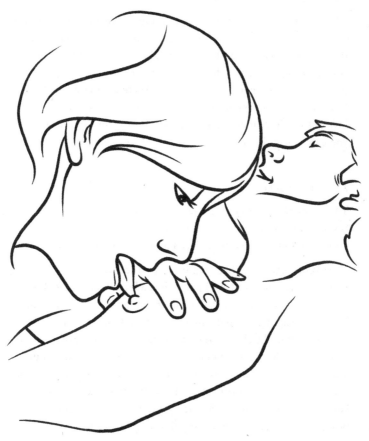

Male nipple stimulation.

A BiGasm

A BiGasm is stimulating two erogenous zones simultaneously to the point of orgasm. It is more intense than a UniGasm, so it's definitely worth exploring.

Ways to create two points of stimulation can be licking the testes while masturbating the penis, sucking on the clitoris while penetrating the anus with a finger (preferably covered with a finger cot), sucking the penis while massaging the testes, or licking the perineum while fingering the clitoris. There are many combinations. Enjoy experimenting on your lover's body, and ask your lover which combinations were most exciting for him or her so you can repeat them.

A TriGasm

The ultimate orgasm is a TriGasm. A female TriGasm is the result of arousing three points of pleasure—the clitoris, G-spot, and anus—simultaneously. Here's how you can do it:

The woman should lie back while her partner lavishes her clitoris with oral pleasure until she has reached a level 8 on her pleasure scale of 1 to 10. Now change course and stimulate her vulva (outside of the vagina) in small circles with your tongue for a few minutes. Return to the clitoris and orally increase her level of pleasure to a 9, almost to the point of no return. At this peak, insert your forefinger palm up into her vagina and find her G-spot, then tap it a few times gently toward her navel. Then, simultaneously stimulate her anus gently with a feather, your pinky, or a vibrator to bring her to a momentous, energy-draining TriGasm.

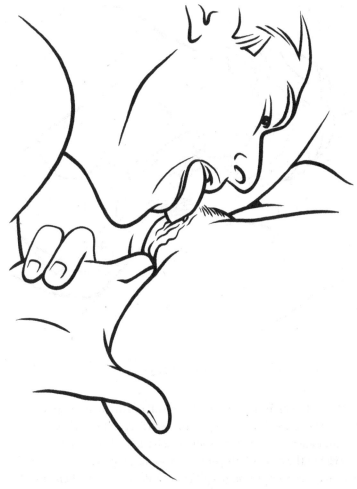

Female TriGasm.

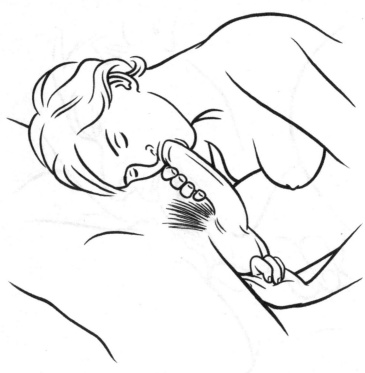

Male TriGasm.

The TriGasm for men is also the result of stimulating three points of pleasure—the penis, the testicles, and the anus—simultaneously. The man should lie back while his partner lavishes the head of his penis with some good oral suction until he reaches a level 8 on his pleasure scale of 1 to 10. Then, use your mouth and tongue to stimulate his testicles for a few minutes while you masturbate his penis with your hand. Return to the penis orally and increase his level of pleasure to a 9, almost to the point of no return. At this peak, fondle his testicles as you continue to orally delight his penis and insert your lubricated forefinger palm up into his anus to find his H-spot (prostate gland), then tap it a few times gently. If all goes well, he'll have an unforgettable, enormous TriGasm.

Believe me when I say that you and your partner will not easily forget experiencing a TriGasm together.

A Blended Orgasm

A blended orgasm is exactly as it sounds, blending more than one orgasm. Start by choosing your favorite orgasm technique (such as oral stimulation on the clitoris for a woman and oral stimulation on the penis for a man). Get aroused to a level 6 on your pleasure scale and then switch to another orgasm technique you enjoy (such as G-spot for a woman and prostate for a guy) and get aroused to a level 7 this time. Switch back to the first technique, raise your arousal level to 8, then go back to the second technique at least three times before reaching a level 10 on your orgasm scale.

Multiple Orgasms

One definition of a multiple orgasm is when you reach one orgasm after another without any rest in between. Another definition is when you have an external orgasm and an internal orgasm simultaneously.

Women can have multiple orgasms, but can men? This is a controversial question, but I say, "Yes." When a man is able to separate ejaculation from his orgasm and he can remain sexually aroused at a very high peak, he can experience multiple orgasms much like a woman can. Multiple orgasms are a learned skill, and just about everyone can be taught to have them, and oral sex is an excellent way to achieve them.

The longest recorded orgasm was 43 seconds with 25 consecutive contractions. The record for the most orgasms by a woman in a single hour is 134.

Sex Juices

Sex is supposed to be wet and juicy; it can also be messy, as sex fluids like saliva, sweat, vaginal secretions, male ejaculate, and even female ejaculate all get mixed up together. Most people enjoy the wetness of sex because it implies that they are having a good time. When a woman's vagina becomes wet, it proves that she is sexually aroused; when a man has pre-ejaculate fluid oozing out of his penis, it means he's getting ready to ejaculate.

It's important to enjoy your own body fluids and to accept your partner's wetness as part of the erotic sexual adventure that goes along with oral sex and lovemaking. The more you know about sex fluids, the more you can enjoy them, so here are the basics on some of the natural fluids we produce when we're having sex.

Semen

Semen is created in the testes, where it takes about 10 weeks for a solitary sperm to reach maturity. The sperm can stay there for about two weeks before it's ready for ejaculation.

Semen contains more than 30 elements, including various vitamins, enzymes, proteins, acids, and salts among others. The consistency of semen can vary depending on diet, medical problems, or even stress. For men to maintain healthy semen, men should avoid smoking, alcohol in excess, coffee, and dairy products because these can make semen taste bitter, and drink plenty of water and eat fresh fruit.

> The approximate amount of semen per ejaculation is 1 to 2 teaspoons. With an average of 7 calories in a teaspoon of semen, it is not fattening. On the contrary, sperm is full of nutrition and protein; however, there's a chance you could catch an STD by swallowing.

Semen can contain all types of bacteria. If you have oral sex without a condom, it's possible to catch an STD, including HIV, even if you don't swallow. Once the semen travels into the stomach, acids in the abdomen can kill the virus. But if there are any open cuts or wounds anywhere ahead of the stomach (including the mouth), there is a risk of infection.

If you want semen to taste its best, men can try this sex shake recipe (formulated by Harley SwiftDeer): 2 teaspoons natural honey, 1 cup of milk, ¼ teaspoon ground cinnamon, ¼ teaspoon ground ginger, ¼ teaspoon ground nutmeg, ¼ teaspoon ground cloves, 1 raw egg. Put all the ingredients into a blender and drink one hour prior to oral sex.

Vaginal Fluids

Healthy vaginal secretion possesses high acidity as a natural resistance to bacteria and helps keep it clean. As discussed in Chapter 2 the vagina is the cleanest orifice in the body because it is self-cleaning and has a perfect pH balance. Vaginal fluids also keep the vagina moist and elastic.

In fact, throughout her monthly cycle, a woman's secretions can change in odor, texture, and color, especially during ovulation and her period. During ovulation, the secretions become much thicker and almost jellylike, and of course during her period her secretions are mixed with blood.

Vaginal secretions can potentially carry bacteria, fungus, and STDs. Unfortunately, antibiotics can cause a nasty discharge because they kill all bacteria, including good bacteria, which the vagina needs to function properly. It's important to learn the difference between healthy vaginal secretions and unhealthy ones. If there is a change in odor, the color turns yellow or green, or the texture is thick and crumbly, she should see a doctor.

Saliva

Saliva comes from the salivary glands located inside of the cheeks and on the bottom of the mouth. These glands secrete slippery fluid every day of our lives.

Some of saliva's benefits include keeping our mouth relatively clean because it contains enzymes that help fight off infections (but brushing our teeth is still essential for oral hygiene). Saliva wets our food so it can push it toward the throat making it easier to swallow. Saliva also helps the tongue to taste and makes for a great natural lubricant when it comes to sex. Plenty of saliva on the head of a man's penis is an erotic way to begin oral sex.

However, as a sexual fluid, saliva can contain viral antibodies and STDs, so be careful not to kiss, lick, or suck someone if you or your partner have a cut or abrasion inside the mouth.

Can Women Ejaculate?

Some women are capable of ejaculating a fluid from their urethra during orgasm. This has been confirmed in several publications such as *The G-Spot* and *Other Recent Discoveries About Human Sexuality,* which offered the theory that a "uterine" orgasm (also known as a G-spot orgasm) can result in female ejaculation.

The fluid expelled looks like watered-down skim milk, and scientists describe it as having little or no color, taste, smell, or residue. The urethra is presumed to be the female prostate, so scientists have compared female ejaculation to male prostatic fluid, except without the sperm. The amount released varies from woman to woman from just a few drops to a gushing of liquid that can soak the sheets.

Any woman can learn to ejaculate, but not all want to. Some women associate it with loss of bladder control and are embarrassed that it might be urine. Although female ejaculate is not urine, it's not as easy to do as men's ejaculation, so not every woman has the desire to invest the time and effort into achieving it. Female ejaculation is associated with contractions of the pubococcygeus muscles (also known as Kegels) during orgasm. Chapter 10 has instructions on how to stimulate the G-spot so a woman can learn to ejaculate if she wants to.

8

Common Oral Sex Mistakes

From orally satisfying all your partner's erogenous zones to complimenting your lover's genitals, there are lots of oral rules you need to know before you can call yourself an oral master or mistress.

In this chapter, you will learn how to avoid some of the most common mistakes women make when handling the penis and men make when exploring the vagina. This chapter will explain why you shouldn't tackle the clitoris too soon and why you shouldn't neglect the testes when pleasuring the penis. You'll find out how to avoid oral pitfalls and make a good impression on your partner with some basic oral etiquette.

Going Down Too Quickly

One of the first mistakes men make is going for the clitoris way too soon. Women really appreciate a slower approach when it comes to sex. They need time to get their juices flowing. Unlike most guys, who can get an erection at a moment's notice, women need to be prepared for sex, even oral sex.

Imagine if you're driving to the airport, you take the freeway to get there because it's quicker and more direct, right? But what if you're taking a drive for pleasure? Why wouldn't you take the scenic route and enjoy the drive? There's no hurry; you can take all the time in the world. Now doesn't that make you feel less pressured, more relaxed, and eager to drive? When it comes to oral sex, work your way there and enjoy the drive.

If in Doubt, Leave It Out

Even though the vagina is self-cleaning, as we talked about earlier in Chapter 2, you still need to know how to keep it that way. If you're good to the vagina, it will return the favor tenfold. Here are some things to remember:

Don't put small objects like marbles inside because they can get out of reach, and then need to be surgically removed. The vagina is a large muscle designed to pull things in, so keep small objects out.

Don't rub or insert anything sugary like honey inside the vagina because it will upset the perfect pH balance that keeps it so clean and healthy. So no Popsicles, chocolate bars, or phallic fruit, either. If you must insert a banana, keep the peel on and put a condom on it first.

Don't insert anything oily because that will cause a nasty vaginal infection. So keep out Vaseline, baby oil, suntan oil, and all cooking oils. Lubricant is all right, as long as it's water soluble.

Don't blow smoke or even air inside the vagina because it can cause an embolism, which is an air bubble that can be fatal if a woman is pregnant.

Don't forget to remove tampons before sex because they can get lodged way up in the vagina and may have to be surgically removed.

Don't have jagged fingernails. Keep them neatly filed because they can cut the vagina.

Don't insert bottles or any other glass, which can shatter.

> Never put anything unsanitary inside the vagina, and that includes unclean fingers.

Don't put alcohol in the vagina. I know some people like to drink and then squirt a little booze into the vagina while giving oral sex. Alcohol will burn the delicate mucous membrane tissue of the vagina. This goes for all kinds of alcohol: wine, whiskey, brandies … everything.

Always remember, if in doubt, leave it out.

Handle with Care

Regardless of what the penis is called when it's hard, the human penis does not have a bone in it. So don't expect him to be hard all the time. The penis is made up of spongy tissue surrounded by a fibrous cover that fills up with blood when aroused, creating an erection.

Most men agree that they like more pressure on their penis than women like on their clitoris, but they'll wince if you squeeze too hard. So take his pride and joy in both hands, wet it with your saliva, and become familiar with it before you take it in your mouth. Don't ever masturbate your man's penis when it's dry; the friction could cause scratches and abrasions. Focus on moving his skin up and down—rather than moving your hand up and down.

Look at his penis admiringly, and feel free to compliment it out loud. Touch it, stroke it, tickle it, pump it between your palms, and rub it all over your body lovingly. A man likes to feel that his partner is enthusiastic about his penis before he surrenders it to his partner's control.

If your man is circumcised, he probably enjoys extra stimulation around the visible scar tissue, located around the head of his penis. Go ahead and add some extra suction around that area as you give him oral sex.

The Issue of Swallowing

If you don't want to swallow, then tell your man before you start giving him oral sex, because he can't read your mind. Furthermore, he may not be able to control himself from climaxing when you're giving him oral sex. It's no fun when you're on the verge of an orgasm and your partner suddenly stops giving you oral sex.

Avoid being uncomfortable by talking to him about your sexual concerns before you become intimate. Voice any fears you may have about gagging or swallowing. Don't ever feel pressured into doing something you don't want to do. A good tip is to agree on a signal he can give you before he's going to climax—such as patting you on the shoulder twice.

Don't Neglect His Testicles

One of the biggest complaints I hear from men is that their lovers neglect their testicles. My advice to men is to remove the hair from their testicles so women will find them more palatable. The penis and testicles are connected, and the penis shaft extends down behind the testicles. Both the penis shaft and the testicles deserve equal attention. It's like putting lipstick on your upper lip and leaving the lower lip without any color.

The testicles are one of the most sensitive parts of the male sexual organ. Touch his testicles delicately, as if you were handling a light bulb. Go ahead and feel, caress, and fondle them, but don't squeeze them too hard. You can also handle the scrotum without touching the testicles; it's less sensitive, but equally erotic and satisfying for the man.

Most men enjoy a wet mouth and talented tongue around their balls, so get used to sucking on the scrotum first and gently tugging on them with your lips, not your teeth. Then take one testicle at a time into your mouth and suck ever so gently, as if you were sucking on a soft-boiled egg, carefully trying not to damage the yolk. After that, suck both testicles at the same time.

Pushing Down

Men should refrain from pushing a woman's head down onto their penis while she's sucking it unless she tells you that she likes you to do that. It turns off some women because it makes them feel like they are being forced to give oral sex.

However, feel free to run your fingers through her hair and gently pull her hair off her face so you can watch her give you oral pleasure. Caress her face tenderly, and give her plenty of encouragement by letting her know how good she makes you feel. The more you tell her that she's skillful, the more she'll want to please you.

Ejaculating Too Quickly

How does it make you feel when your sexy lover goes down on you? She begins to lick the head of your penis with her luscious tongue, parts her lips and takes your shaft deep into her mouth, and then suddenly it's all over—you couldn't hold back and you came much sooner than you wanted. Some men say it makes them feel inadequate as a lover; others just get mad at themselves. Premature ejaculation can happen to anyone, but if you want to avoid the embarrassment, here are some precautions you can take:

- If you haven't had sex in a long time, masturbate about four hours before your planned encounter.

- If you are getting oral sex and you feel like you're going to climax, ask your partner to stop. Then give her oral sex for a while.

- You can squeeze the base of your penis when you feel like you're going to climax too early.

Watch Your Teeth

When teeth brush up against a penis or a clitoris, it will spoil the moment and possibly the rest of the night. Most of the time, if your teeth come in contact with your partner's skin, you probably won't realize it, but your partner will.

For her: The first step to keeping your teeth off his penis is to be aware that you have sharp weapons in your mouth. The next step is to be sure your jaw is open relatively wide when giving oral sex so your teeth won't come in contact with your partner's genitals. In the heat of passion, to avoid accidental scraping, wrap your lips around your teeth. Ladies, this is especially important when you are deep-throating your man. If you are still unable to control your teeth, another alternative is to cover them with plastic teeth guards that come in over-the-counter teeth-whitening kits.

For him: The worst thing a guy can do is to chew on the clitoris. Start licking the clitoris gently with the tip of your tongue. As you feel her thrusting forward, keep your upper lip over your teeth to protect her from getting bitten, and continue licking with rhythmic strokes. She will continue to push her lower body toward you in her desire for more pressure, and all you have to do is to continue licking until she pushes you away.

Not Being Prepared

There's nothing worse than having a dry mouth when you are trying to satisfy your partner orally, so try to have a glass of water nearby so you can take a discreet sip whenever you need it.

If you're feeling adventurous, add some ice cubes to use on your lover for some sensual foreplay. The same goes for a towel or tissues to wipe away body fluids. Keep them close by so you don't have to jump up as soon as you and your partner have climaxed. Some people prefer the taste of flavored lubricants to the natural taste of their partner's genitals, so keep these handy if you're going to use them.

It's a hassle, and bad etiquette, to get up in the middle of adult play to get a glass of water or even to go to the bathroom. It breaks the mood. Go to the bathroom before you make love. Open up your condom, get out your sex toys, and prepare everything you need before you get all worked up. Better still, go to the bathroom together and take a shower or bubble bath before oral sex so you both feel squeaky clean.

What Not to Say

When you're giving or receiving oral sex, here are some things you definitely don't want to say:

Don't talk about problems. It's a sure way to kill the mood, and it lets your partner know you're not turned on.

Don't talk about your body negatively. Don't blurt out, "I wish my stomach was flatter." Worse still, don't insult your partner's body.

Don't compare your partner to anyone else you have slept with.

Don't call her a whore or anything else that is derogatory, unless you both discuss it beforehand. Some women enjoy hearing sexually graphic language while they are giving fellatio. So if your lover gives you permission to talk to her like a whore, then by all means, go for it—just don't assume it's okay.

Don't ask a woman if she came. You should know whether she did or not by her body language.

Don't ask your lover to answer an awkward question like, "Am I the best lover you've ever had?" especially if you can't handle the truth.

Don't say "Stop" when you mean "Go," and don't say "No" when you mean "Yes."

Don't negatively express directions to your lover on how you like to receive oral sex. It's okay to say, "I love it when you lick the head gently with your tongue," but it's not okay to say, "Why don't you lick the head more?"

Don't get carried away during oral sex and say something you'll regret later like, "I love you," if you don't mean it. Instead, you can say, "I love making love to you," or "I love being with you," but don't ever play with someone's emotions.

There are two very powerful words you can use in bed that will turn on your partner. The first one is "yes," and the second is his or her name.

Common Turn-Offs

Some things to keep in mind before you get down to business are:

Don't attack your lover's sense of smell by pouring on too much perfume or cologne, especially around your genitals. There's nothing sexier than the aroma of a clean body. Even if it cost you a small fortune, go easy on the perfume—it tastes bad, it can linger on the sheets and furniture, and it can even cause allergies.

Don't put talcum powder on your genitals before oral sex because it clumps up when you sweat, looks yucky, and tastes horrible.

Don't use depilatory cream to remove pubic hair just before getting oral sex. The skin is very sensitive after using depilatory cream, and even a wet tongue can result in a burning sensation. The odor also lingers for several hours. It's best to use the cream the night before.

Don't leave a hickey as your calling card on your lover unless he or she asks you to.

9

Oral Sex Options

Now that you know some basic oral sex techniques, it's time to turn up the heat with various oral sex options. By the time you've finished this chapter, you will be well on your way to becoming an oral master or mistress.

In this chapter, you'll discover how to incorporate some common household items into foreplay and why sex toys have therapeutic value. You'll have the opportunity to expand your sexual horizon by sharing your sexual fantasies and role-playing with your lover. Enjoy legendary aphrodisiacs, and for the truly adventurous, embark on some back door fun.

Positions for His Pleasure

Receiving oral sex feels great in pretty much any position you choose, and there are lots to select from. Some positions make you feel more outgoing than others, and each position stimulates you differently. Try new positions and locations if you want to maintain excitement in your sex life. Here's some to get you started.

Lying Back

Guys love this position since all they have to do is lie on their back with a pillow under their head and another pillow under their buttocks. This position can be accomplished on a bed, a couch, or the floor. It offers easy access to his penis, testicles, and anus and allows him to lie back totally relaxed. Ladies, you can rest yourself in between his legs, on your stomach so you have a bird's-eye view of his entire genital area.

Begin by taking his penis in your hands and licking the head in circular motions as you maintain eye contact with him. Apply plenty of saliva to make his penis wet and slippery. Next, wrap your lips tightly around the head of his penis, and use your mouth as a vacuum (not an industrial vacuum—more like a handheld vacuum), by lavishing him with ample suction.

Now you are well on your way to giving him a memorable blow job. Remember to make sounds of pleasure as you orally delight him, use your hands as an extension of your mouth, and be sure to stimulate his testicles.

Turnaround

In this position, the guy continues to lay back, but you get to sit on his chest, facing away from him. If you lift your buttocks up slightly, it will give him an erotic visual of you, while you have a new angle for orally pleasing him. If you suffer from the gag reflex, this angle will help lessen it. It's also a great position for you to stimulate his prostate area.

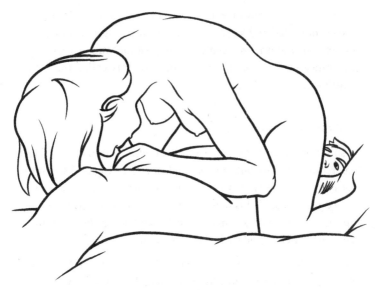

Turnaround position.

Knees Up

Remaining on his back, the guy lifts his knees to his chest, and places his feet on his lover's shoulders while she kneels between his legs. His penis, testicles, and anus are on complete display, giving her easy access to orally lavish them all.

Straddling

Now she is lying on her back, and he straddles her face putting his knees on either side of her face so his penis hovers over her mouth. He can do this facing her or facing away from her. Either way, she gets a good angle for some deep-throating.

Communicate in advance if he should remain still while you move your head and hands or if he can thrust his penis in and out of your mouth. This angle is also great for orally pleasuring the testicles and the anus. (We'll expand on this, called analingus, a little later in this chapter.)

Doggie Pose

It's nice to know that this position is conducive to more than just intercourse. It's actually a great angle for receiving oral sex, both for men and women. Let's focus on his pleasure first as he gets into doggie pose on his hands and knees with his legs spread apart. By drawing his penis back between his legs, he can now be lavishly licked and sucked by his partner.

You can also bend over a bed, chair, or even a table and use the furniture as leverage, instead of putting all the weight on your hands and knees. If you want to be even more comfortable, just lie down on your stomach with your legs spread wide apart. Your partner can still get a mouthful of your penis and testes. Remember, variety is the spice of life, and that includes oral sex positions.

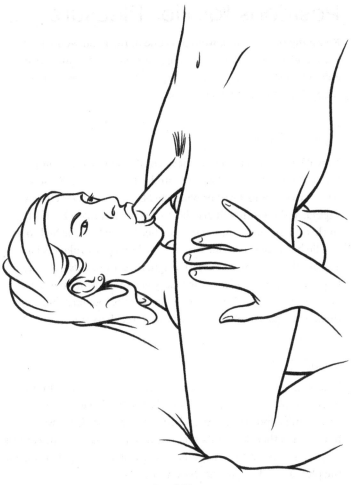

Straddling.

Positions for Her Pleasure

Receiving oral sex for a woman is one of the great wonders of the world. Getting into various oral sex positions is an added enjoyment she will be only too happy to engage in, especially when she is the focus of attention.

Lying Back

Now it's the lady's turn to lie back comfortably with a soft pillow under her head and another under her buttocks. Raising her pelvis with a pillow will provide the best access to her clitoris, vagina, and anus. It will also help alleviate strain on his neck. In this classic position, she spreads her legs flat on the bed so he can lie between them. She can use her hands to stroke his hair and gently guide his head in the right direction. Guys, feel free to put your arms under her legs so you can draw her buttocks even closer to you. Don't squeeze her cheeks too hard, but spread them apart gently. Now enjoy giving as much as you get.

Legs Up

Still lying on her back, she raises both legs and rests them on her lover's shoulders. This position is one that gives her sexual organs full exposure and even better oral access. Some women like it when their lover lifts their buttocks up high, but be careful because it can put a strain on her back as it arches up. For others, the pleasure outweighs the discomfort.

Knees Up

Remaining on her back, she bends and raises her knees so she can rest them on his chest. Now she can surrender herself to his mouth and tongue.

Straddling

In this position, ladies can wear a G-string, and pull it to one side to tease him first. She straddles his face by squatting or kneeling over him.

Facing him or turning the other way, either way, it's a great oral sex position for the woman because she can control the pressure and tempo of the pleasure she is getting. By lifting and lowering the vagina, grinding the hips, and tilting the pelvis, she's in control.

Doggie Pose

This position is particularly popular with women who are sexually uninhibited. Licking her from behind while she's in doggie pose gives the man great access to her vagina and anus. Men find this position one of the most erotic, and women love the stimulation they get from this angle.

She can try bending over a bed or some furniture and using it as leverage instead of putting all the weight on her hands and knees. For more comfort, she can just lie down on her stomach with her legs spread wide apart. This position is great because you can stimulate her clitoris while lavishing oral sex on and in her vagina. Ladies, be prepared to reach your climax sooner than you think!

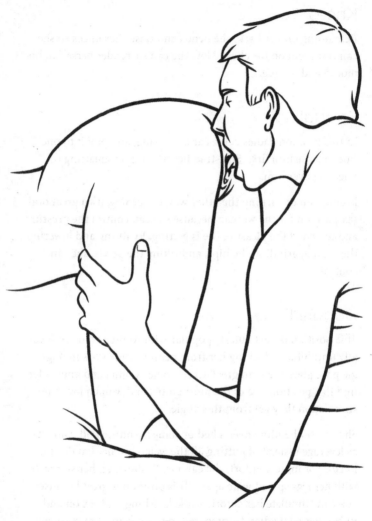

Doggie pose.

Sitting

Ladies, sit upon your throne and prepare to be orally pampered. Actually, you can sit anywhere—on the edge of the bed, on the kitchen counter, or even on the tumble dryer—which is best when it's on spin cycle. Your lover will kneel or crouch in front of you, and he'll either hold your legs up over his head or let them rest on his shoulders. Either way, you'll be the receiver of oral delights.

Standing

This is a hot fantasy for both sexes. Ladies, this is your opportunity to dominate your man. Stand up against a wall or counter and ask your lover to kneel down before you. Lift one leg and put your foot on his shoulder. Now hold on to his head and guide it toward your vagina while you give him plenty of encouragement.

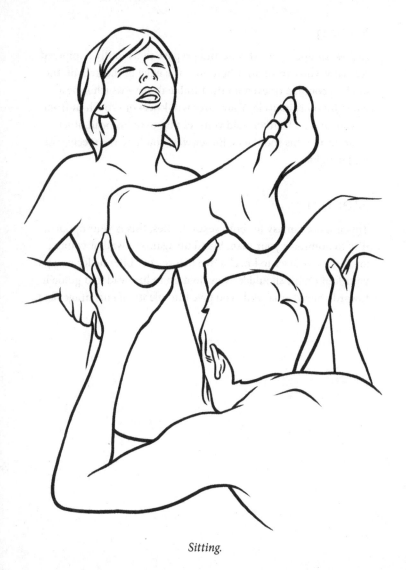

Sitting.

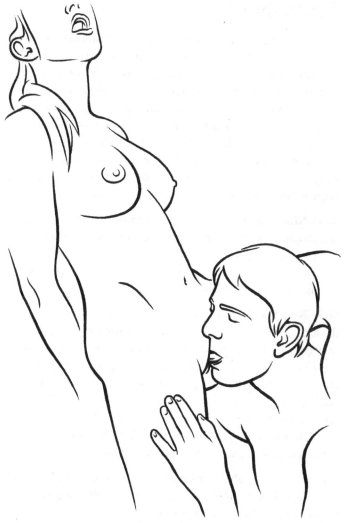

Standing.

Sixty-Nine

The sixty-nine position is a great one for mutual oral sex. First you have to decide who is going to be on top—my suggestion is the lighter one of the two of you should be on his or her hands and knees over the other. Admittedly, it can be distracting when you're trying to give oral sex and you're receiving it at the same time. Be careful not to get too aggressive with your lover's genitals in this position. If you have trouble keeping rhythm or concentrating on giving while you're receiving, you can stay in the sixty-nine position and masturbate your partner while she or he is giving you oral sex. Here are a couple more options:

Sixty-Nine Sideways: This position is most comfortable for people who are of ample weight, which includes pregnant women. Lie down on your side, your mouth facing your partner's genitals. Because your head is in between your partner's legs, you can use each other's thighs as a pillow.

Sixty-Nine Standing: This is only for the truly athletic, not for the weak at heart. Men, lift up your lover and spin her around so her vagina is in your face and her head is down between your legs so she can put her mouth around your penis. Now hold on to her nice and tight because you don't want to drop her on her head. This position is as advanced as you can get, and it's also very playful. Just give each other a few good licks and then put her back down the right way up. Though it's not a great position to reach orgasm, I guarantee it will be memorable.

Talk to each other about which positions you enjoy the most and why you find them more exciting than others. By changing positions during oral sex, the receiver experiences a variety of feelings according to the angle.

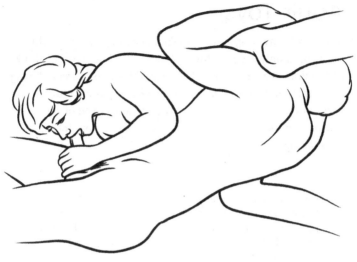

Sixty-nine sideways.

Change Locations

You don't want to always make love in the same old place, in the same old position at the same old time—boring, boring, boring! There's no better way to keep your love life fresh than to keep your lover guessing, "I wonder where we'll make love next." Change where you have oral sex as often as you can. Whether you live in a house or an apartment, there are several options to choose from. Christen every room in your home by having an orgasm in each one.

Adult Toys

A sex toy is anything you use to enhance foreplay or sex. The most commonly used sex toy is the vibrator. Many people think of vibrators as a woman's tool to be used for solo pleasure during masturbation. However, many men enjoy the stimulation of a vibrator on their genitals, testicles, and anus. And of course couples can incorporate vibrators and other sex toys into their lovemaking.

> Don't forget to clean your sex toys with soap and water as you would anything else you use regularly. You can also practice putting condoms on the vibrators and dildos for fun.

I believe sex toys have therapeutic value because they can help people overcome inhibitions, add a wonderful source of variety, and can spice up a predictable lovemaking session. They can also take performance pressure off the man and help both sexes to reach orgasms more readily. And of course the sex toy can keep on going and going as long as it has working batteries.

Today there are hundreds of vibrators and dildos in all shapes and sizes. I recommend couples go sex toy shopping together so they can each pick out one sex toy they want to take home with them. Whether you visit a sex toy shop or purchase your adult toys on the Internet, you'll have something new and exciting to add to your sexual repertoire.

> Never use a sex toy for the vagina that has been inserted into the anus, and never share your sex toys with anyone else.

By combining vibrators and dildos with oral sex, you can fantasize that you're having sex with more than one person and add extra stimulation at the same time.

For her: You are lying back, enjoying the way your lover is licking your clitoris and he's slowly penetrating your vagina with a dildo at the same time. You can fantasize that you have two lovers; you can experience a clitoral orgasm and a G-spot orgasm simultaneously and enjoy the uninhibited pleasure of surrendering yourself to your partner.

For him: Your lover is straddled above you in the sixty-nine position as she is giving you a phenomenal blow job. Your erect penis is filling her mouth—then she takes a vibrator and places it in the middle of your testicles. You are experiencing suction around your penis, vibration in the center of your testicles, then … she adds a vibrating butt plug to the opening of your anus. The feeling is unbearably good, and you can't hold back anymore. You're in sex toy heaven.

Back Door Fun

Many people wince at the thought of anal play because they consider the anus an exit, not an entrance, and certainly not a lickable source of power-packed pleasure. For others, though, rimming, or analingus (kissing, caressing, or penetrating the anal opening with a tongue) is an orgasmic experience. Because many consider the anus taboo, it can heighten the erotica both for the giver and receiver. The anus is surrounded by sensitive nerve endings, which is another reason why it can take you to the point of no return.

Great oral sex can include stimulating the anus with a feather, vibrator, pinky, or tongue. Here are some anal tips for the anal adventurer:

- The easiest position for analingus is doggie pose.

- Start by gently kissing your partner's butt cheeks.

- Using the flat of your tongue, lick your partner's perineum (located between the man's testicles and his anus or the woman's vaginal opening and her anus) all the way to your partner's anus.

- With the tip of your tongue, lightly lick around the anal button in circular motions.

- With a pointy tongue, give your partner's anus an in-and-out massage.

As a word of caution, you should know that the anus is not as clean as the vagina. In fact, it is filled with bacteria so oral-anal contact is not a safe one. Unprotected, it can transmit viruses that include HIV, hepatitis, herpes, and warts. Always use a barrier such as a dental dam or even transparent food wrap when engaging in analingus.

Have fun!

10

How to Rock Her World

In this chapter, you'll get the facts on what women need to be fully aroused. You'll learn how to stimulate all her senses, get the lowdown on how to identify your lover's erogenous zones with your tongue, learn tips on facial intercourse and shrimping, and understand why enthusiasm is so important. You will feel like a hero when you discover her G-spot and help her achieve multiple orgasms. This chapter will help create the most memorable sex of her life.

Sensational Sex

All the senses come into play for a woman to experience phenomenal oral sex. Taking the time to stimulate all of them before heading south is a sure-fire way to get her relaxed, aroused, and ready for great oral sex.

If you don't use one of your five senses during lovemaking, you miss out on 20 percent of pleasure.

What Smells Good

Our most powerful sense is smell, because smell receptors in the nose are directly wired to the limbic center of the brain. It controls our sex drive, emotions, and sensual memories. So a smell can arouse us, trigger an emotion, or evoke a memory.

The number one reason you choose a lover above anything else is because you love the way they smell. Our natural pheromones are how we attract our mates. These pheromones come from our sweat glands that are attached to our hair follicles. So wherever there is hair, there are pheromones: in our scalp, under our arms, and in our pubic hair.

If you want to rock her world, you need to know how to heighten her sense of smell. Women are attracted to the aroma of musk, orange-blossom, and sandalwood, many of which are ingredients found in men's cologne. So before buying any, ask her what kind of men's fragrance turns her on. Food aromas that turn women on include melon, chocolate, oranges, and fresh bread. You can also stimulate her sense of smell with scented candles, fresh flowers, or incense.

What Looks Good

We all know how visual guys are, which is why they love to see their ladies wear sexy lingerie. But don't underestimate your woman's sense of sight. She wants to be stimulated visually just as much as you do. Women love to see their man perfectly groomed, so always try to look your best for your lover. Arouse her sense of sight by lowering the lights or candlelight and give her oral sex in front of a mirror. Some women love watching erotica, too—I have a feeling you won't object if she wants to watch an adult movie with you.

What Sounds Good

Nothing stimulates the sense of hearing better than some erotic talk. Whisper lots of compliments in her ear and tell her how you plan to seduce her orally. Don't forget to use her name. Other sensual sound stimulants are a crackling fireplace, sensual music, nature sounds, and even the sounds of other people making love. You can always record yourselves having sex and then play it back the next time you make love.

What Feels Good

Slowly, sensuously undress your lover and caress, kiss, and lick every part of her body as you peel off her clothes. Give her oral sex on satin sheets; caress her body with different fabrics like feathers, silk, velvet, or leather. Cover her body in massage oil, lotion, or powder. Just don't touch that TV remote, because she should be the one and only focus of your attention.

What Tastes Good

Prepare some erotic finger foods in advance of your sexual activity, such as fruits like strawberries, bananas, mangoes, and juicy oranges to dip in melted chocolate and whipped cream. Feed each other and lick each other's fingers before moving down for oral pleasure.

Use edible lotions, potions, and lubricants, but remember to only put these foods and products on your lover, not inside her vagina because it has a perfect pH balance that should not be upset.

Lick Her from Head to Toe

How many times have you heard that women want foreplay, and plenty of it? Well, I'm here to confirm that it's true. We need to be prepared for sex to get our natural juices flowing. One of the most effective ways to get your woman in the mood for love, especially oral love, is for you to stimulate her erogenous zones. Women are covered in erogenous zones (places on the body that, when stimulated, give pleasure and lead to sexual arousal) from head to toe. It's your job to discover her primary erogenous zones and then work her up to a sexual frenzy.

The best way to discover your lover's erogenous zones is to kiss and lick her from her head to her toes in slow motion. Don't leave out any areas, especially if you see an imperfection like a mole or a scar. Go ahead kiss the flaw on her body. It will help her relax and give her more sexual confidence. Now ask your lover to rate her erogenous zones on a pleasure scale from 1 to 10 with 10, being orgasmic. You can use your tongue to help her discover new, exquisite zones of pleasure. Wet your tongue; use it dry; try circular motions; sweeping motions; and spell your name on your lover's body. This licking will prepare you for giving her great oral sex.

Facial Intercourse

Kissing is so intimate and erotic that I like to call it facial intercourse. The way you kiss also reveals a lot about the way you give oral sex. Most women love to be kissed for at least five minutes. Pay attention to her face before you go below the belt. Add some variety to your standard kissing technique. Start by brushing her hair back off her face and gently massage her scalp as you cover her face with baby kisses.

Then lick her upper and lower lips with the tip of your tongue. Now run your tongue over her teeth. Wrap your lips around her tongue and suck deeply and gently, then dart your tongue in and out of her mouth and let her tongue search the inside of your mouth. Your journey has only just begun.

There are lots of different kinds of kisses: slow, quick, wet, dry, long, etc. Don't take the art of kissing for granted. Add variety to your kissing technique and make it last for a minimum of 12 seconds.

Explore Her Whole Body

Now that your tongue is all warmed up, it's time to explore all her erogenous zones. Remember to get feedback from her on which ones turn her on the most. You don't need to write them down, but you do need to remember the ones that are rated 8 and above.

- Kiss her ear lobes gently. If she rates it a high number, continue to kiss, lick, and suck on them. She'll start to turn to putty in your hands.

- Massage her neck and shoulders with your fingertips, and follow with quick flicks of your tongue.

- The fingers are especially sensitive. Spread two fingers apart at a time and lick in between them with a pointy tongue.

- Surprisingly, the armpits are an erogenous zone for many women—so give them a lick and find out if your lover enjoys it.

- The breasts are an obvious hot spot, and they should be kissed and fondled gently. Avoid contact with the nipples until after you've kissed and licked the underside of her breasts. A common criticism I hear from women is that men are too rough with their nipples. If you start out by kissing, licking, then sucking the nipples softly, you can't go wrong.

- A woman's belly is all too often neglected, so here's your chance to lightly tickle her belly, followed by light circular licks with your tongue.

- Inside the thighs are especially responsive to a nice wet tongue—tease her inner thighs without touching the genitals.

- Ask her to turn over and lick the back of her neck, then blow your warm breath on her nape and shoulders.

- Licking up and down the spine can create goose bumps, so wet your whistle and go for it.

- Her buttocks are just aching to be massaged, kissed, and licked.

- Slide your tongue up and down the back of her thighs— if your tongue gets tired, alternate kisses and licks.

You've invested some quality time exploring your lover's feminine curves. You're on your way to "rocking her world"—the more you tease her, the more excited she'll become and the quicker she'll climax.

Shrimping

Before you focus on her vagina, there's one more area that needs particular attention. Her toes! Having her toes licked is a major turn-on for some women. Be sure you give every toe equal attention by licking in between each one and then sucking them individually. This is a popular fetish known as shrimping. It's fittingly named because the toes on your feet resemble a row of shrimp.

Show Your Enthusiasm

It cannot be stressed enough that enthusiasm is more important than technique. Fortunately for you, this book will help you with both. Women love a man who is enthusiastic, especially when it comes to giving her oral sex. The more you let her know how much you love going down on her, the better. Tell her that she tastes delicious, she smells great, and her vagina looks beautiful. Let her know that you could give her oral sex all night long, if that's what she wanted.

Use the Alphabet

This technique will take your lover to the point of no return and back again. Just let her know that she is going to be the receiver of pleasure and you are going to be the giver. I hope you can remember the alphabet because you're going to spell it out on her vagina with your tongue. If all goes according to plan, she'll have the big "O" before you even get to O.

The best position for this is any of the contented female positions (from Chapter 9) where she is lying comfortably on her back with a pillow behind her head and another under her buttocks.

1. Start by covering her vagina with your entire mouth. This lets her know she's in for a treat. Incidentally, I recommend that you end each oral sex session with the same loving ritual by covering her entire vagina with your entire mouth for a few seconds.

2. Now begin tracing the capital letter A with the tip of your tongue from the top of her clitoris all the way down to the opening of her vagina. Make your tongue flat and wide when you cross the letter A.

3. The letter B has a few more curves in it, which will stimulate different parts of her vagina. Use a firm tongue stroke to circle the top of the B around her clitoris, inadvertently flicking it before you tongue the second circle.

4. Continue to slide and twist your tongue around her vulva as you spell the rest of the alphabet.

Use your tongue in different ways, alternating from up and down, side to side, small and big circles, soft and firm, quick and slow, pointed and flat. Have a good time exercising your tongue and pleasing your mate. I'm betting she won't let you finish the alphabet. Incidentally, you can also trace numbers on her vagina.

Find Her G-Spot

The G-spot, which I like to refer to as the goddess spot because it makes a woman feel like a goddess when it's stimulated, is not a myth—every woman has one, though not every woman has experienced a G-spot orgasm. Even though the G-spot is about two inches inside the vagina, it can still be stimulated during oral sex.

Here is the best way to find and stimulate her goddess spot. But before you begin, be sure your lover is well lubricated either naturally or from using some commercial lubricants like Wet or Astroglide (available at most pharmacies).

1. Begin by resting your thumb on her clitoris while inserting the middle finger of your prominent hand in a "come here" motion into her vagina, palm up.

2. Imagine there is a clock on the inside of your partner's vagina and you are stroking from 6 o'clock (at the bottom of her vaginal opening) to 12 o'clock (her G-spot). Use long strokes, creating an energetic circuit between your thumb and finger.

3. The goddess spot is about the size of a dime. It will feel different to the rest of the tissue inside the vagina. It will feel like it has ridges on it, much like corduroy material or the roof of your mouth.

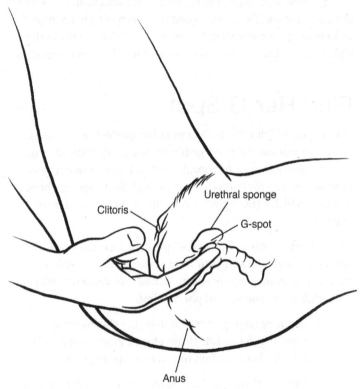

Finding her G-spot.

By stimulating her G-spot and lavishing her clitoris with oral sex, you will help your lover achieve multiple orgasms—a clitoral orgasm and a goddess orgasm simultaneously—and guys, you will be a hero. So follow carefully:

1. Pull back the clitoral hood.

2. Lick the clitoris, alternating with short strokes directly on the clitoris and long strokes that start at the vaginal opening and end at the clitoris. Do this until she reaches a level 8 on her pleasure scale of 1 to 10. Remember, if she reaches a 10, you'll have to start all over again. Ask her to let you know when she's reached a level 8. Depending on your partner's personal sexual cycle, her response could take anywhere from 2 to 15 minutes. It has nothing to do with your performance.

3. Move your tongue away from the clitoris and stimulate the entire vaginal opening in circular tongue motions, from smaller to larger circles, licking every inch of her vaginal opening. Do this for a couple minutes only.

4. Go back to stimulating her clitoris with short and long strokes until she reaches a level 9 on her pleasure scale. Be sure she doesn't get carried away.

5. Now slip the middle finger of your prominent hand inside her vagina, palm up so you can find the goddess spot. Meanwhile, continue to lick her clitoris with only short strokes.

6. Once your finger is on top of her G-spot, tap it toward the belly button, still maintaining oral stimulation on her clitoris.

7. Now you continue to tap her G-spot and lick her clitoris rhythmically until she reaches her multiple orgasms.

This technique is one that will leave your lover exhausted, exhilarated, and extremely satisfied.

Stimulation of the clitoris (the primary sexual organ) and the breasts (the secondary sexual organ) at the same time can send women to orgasmic bliss. Do this in the 69 position with your penis in between her breasts instead of her mouth while you lick her clitoris.

11

How to Rock His World

In this chapter, you'll learn advanced oral sex techniques that will make you a fellatio aficionado. You'll discover how to become a sex slave one minute and a dominatrix the next. Find out why men enjoy oral sex in the morning and how you can leave a lasting impression he'll never forget. You'll also be taught all about his H-spot, and how to stimulate it so he can experience multiple orgasms.

The Eyes Have It

Most men will confess that erotic stimulation is about 70 percent visual and 30 percent physical. That should give you a clue as to what to do to rock his world.

Do anything you can do to be different, better, more creative, and adventurous, and don't be afraid to initiate sex, especially oral sex. Because men tend to become turned on visually, you can do a lot to bring a man to climax simply by using your body in imaginative ways.

Bear in mind that men are not biologically pro-
grammed to be with one lover. Gain the edge
over a man's natural tendencies to play the field
by keeping your sex life interesting. If you want a
monogamous man, you need to make it happen.

Dress for Success

Since men are so strongly stimulated visually, the first step is
to dress in sexy lingerie, like low-cut bras, suspender hose, a
G-string or transparent panties, thigh highs, and other assorted
lingerie for your man's enjoyment. Don't forget the high-heeled
stilettos. There's nothing more exciting for a man (no matter
what age he is) than when he finds his date has stockings and a
garter belt under her dress.

Experience the allure of dressing in stockings and titillating lingerie for yourself and discover how sexy you
feel when you wear them. He, of course, will love it.

Do a Striptease

The ultimate fantasy for a man is to watch his lover do a striptease for him. Your interpretation of the striptease depends
solely on your mood and the image you wish to project—from
artfully subtle to elegant, sexy, and chic, to lusty, wild, and
X-rated. Your outfit is a provocative prelude to an ultra-hot com-
ing attraction … you!

If you're still wrestling with shyness, rent some movies like *9½ Weeks, True Lies, Striptease,* or *Showgirls,* and see how it's done. Once you get over the first-time jitters, you'll get as involved in the eroticism of the striptease as he will. Try it, you'll like it, and he'll love it!

Choose some music you can move to (Chapter 4 has some suggestions). Stand in front of your lover, maintaining eye contact with him. Rub your hands all over your fully clad body in slow motion and give him a seductive little smile. Then remove your dress and let it fall to the floor, step back, and let him admire your legs and body encased in the nylons and lingerie. Turn around so he can appreciate your rear framed by the garter belt and stockings. Bend over and wiggle your butt teasingly. Turn back toward him, and slink your way between his legs. Don't take off your shoes, even for oral sex, because they complete the outfit.

Ripping Your Clothes Off

Let your lover tear your clothes off of you and adoringly ravage you. From your blouse to your underwear, pick out pieces you know will turn him on and just let him rip them off. If the material is too thick, cut it in strategic places so they tear off more easily.

Do a Photo Shoot

To your lover, you are a centerfold model, so ask him to take some photos of you partially clad or completely nude. This visual treat can really get the juices flowing and rev up your sex life.

Cleavage Fornication

Use your breasts to their full advantage. Hang your breasts over him and push them on his face, then down the rest of his body until you are kneeling on the floor with your breasts at the same level as his penis. This is guaranteed to get the proverbial rise out of him. Unzip his pants, if they are not already off, and place his penis between your breasts. Remove your bra or ask him to unsnap your bra for you as you continue to push your breasts together (this works no matter what size they are) and lift your breasts up and down with his penis tightly packed in the middle between them. This is called cleavage fornication, and men love it.

Become His Sex Slave

Let him know you want to be his sex slave for one hour (or more) and that you'll do anything he wants. Be open to fulfilling all of his sexual desires. I pretty much guarantee visual delights leading to oral sex will be part of his pleasure plan. To add to this fantasy, refer to your lover as "Master." Remember that oral sex is adult play, so have fun with it.

Deep-Throating

Most men will want to straddle their partner's face and penetrate their mouth with their penis for a deep-throat experience. If you are not adverse to this, lie down and throw your head back so you can open up your mouth and throat. Be sure you have plenty of saliva in your mouth, breathe through your nose, and then try sliding his penis down your throat as far as it will go. In case you start to feel yourself gagging, have some lubricant ready to put on your hand so that it's wet, then take a hold of the base of his penis and use your hand as an extension of your mouth by rubbing it up and down to the same tempo as your mouth.

Another deep-throat technique is to twist your head in a circular motion, which requires more effort (and enthusiasm) for you to turn your head and neck while sucking his penis deeply.

Tea-Bagging

If deep-throating is not your bag, then you might consider tea-bagging. It's a term often used by gay men to describe dipping testicles into an eager and open mouth. As his sex slave, you can lie obediently beneath him and maneuver his testicles into your mouth. Start by running your tongue around each ball, licking it slowly, then change the rhythm to a faster, more intense licking, being careful to watch those teeth, until you are ready for the tea-bagging ceremony.

Dip one testicle at a time into your mouth, and remember his balls are delicate. Suck on it as if you were savoring the flavor of a ripe plum, draining the juice out of it, without biting into it. If you think you can handle it, try to dip both of his balls into your mouth and lick with your tongue as you suck with your mouth. If your jaw can only stay wide open for a few moments, that will be enough to impress him so he'll always remember it, and you.

Dominate Him

If you've ever wanted a man to worship you and treat you like a goddess, you need to know how to unleash the tigress within you. I believe every woman has a dominatrix inside of her that wants to come out and play. Be bold and playful so you can become the confident and dominant woman you were created to be.

Dress up in your most erotic yet dominant outfit. Leather boots, a latex mini skirt, and black top are perfect. The outfit will help you get into character. Tell your man you want him totally naked before you. Make him bend over and spank his butt with your hairbrush, saying, "You've been a very bad boy so you have to be punished." Demand that he suck on your breasts, spread your labia, and lick your clit. Then tell him that if he doesn't do it well, he won't get a blow job. Be a bitch.

Once you have him in a place of submission, change your character. Go from aggressive to gentle. Hold him, kiss him, and tell him he's been a good boy. Take him to a comfortable bed or couch and have him lay down on his back.

Now tell him that the only way he's going to get a blow job is if he begs you for it. Just watch how aroused he gets with this kind of talk and role-playing. Most men enjoy some kind of female authority in the bedroom. When he says the word *please* you can circle your tongue around the head of his penis and gently tug on his testicles simultaneously. This is also a great way to get him to talk erotically to you. Encourage him to tell you what he likes and how he likes it. Alternatively, you can demand that he describe what you are doing to him in graphic detail. To heighten the sexual excitement, maintain eye contact with him while you do the following:

- Lick his raphe (the seam that runs along the underside of the penis) with the flat of your tongue. Then press your tongue flat on his frenulum with his penis balancing on your tongue and hold it still for a few moments.

- Put your finger (palm up) inside his mouth while you slide his penis slowly into your mouth, pulling him in with your lips, moving back and forth. Suck him deeper with each forward motion.

- Change your rhythm from long, slow sucking to short, fast-milking action, making lots of slurping noises as you suck. Hold onto his hips or butt and pull him toward you as you increase the pace.

- Shake and wiggle his penis in your mouth as you create a vacuum suction with your lips.

- Pump his penis shaft with one (lubricated) hand while you concentrate on sucking the glans with short, intense motions.

The more he begs you, the more you should fellate him.

More mature men need greater pressure to get any specific sensation, while younger men mostly enjoy a lighter touch.

Morning Glory

It's a fact that most men wake up with an erection in the morning because they need to empty their bladder, but it's also a fact that men's sexual hormone levels are higher in the morning, which means they are ready for sexual activity. Even if you're not a morning person, give him a treat once in a while so he can go to work with a smile on his face and a swing in his walk.

When you first wake up, your mouth can feel as dry as a rock. If you drink something or suck on a candy, it will get the saliva flowing. There's nothing sexier than surprising your man with a morning blow job. Slide under the sheets and nestle in between his legs, where you can manipulate his penis with your hands and mouth. Start by caressing him with your fingertips by walking them up and down his shaft and around the tip. Then blow your warm breath up and down his penis, and around his testicles and anus area. Brush your hair against his penis and stroke your face with it. Hold the base as you taste him by licking around the coronal ridge. Flick your tongue back and forth over the frenulum. Then create a seal around his glans with your mouth as you let your tongue dance around it. As you do this, make light humming sounds to give him some extra vibration. This is a sure way to get him to return the favor, and maybe even make you breakfast in bed.

His Inner H-Spot

The man's equivalent of a woman's G-spot is his prostate gland, which I like to call his "H-spot" for hero spot. I've been told by men that when they reach a climax through prostate gland stimulation combined with oral sex, it is an unforgettable, mind-blowing multi-orgasmic experience. But lacking a vagina, there is no direct route to it. You can reach it in two ways, however.

One is by using your finger or dildo to reach into his anus—this is a little tricky, so be sure he is willing to tell you when it is "feeling good." His H-spot is about one to two inches inside the anus.

The prostate gland is about the size of a walnut. It surrounds the urethra and is at the neck of the bladder. This gland produces the majority of the ejaculatory fluid expelled in semen.

Before you start, be sure to lubricate your finger and then gently ease it into him, keeping in mind that just an inch or so of penetration will get you to his H-spot. If you use your finger to reach inside him, buy some latex finger cots at the drugstore, which are ideal for this purpose. They can be easily lubricated and just as easily discarded after use to prevent the potential spread of bacteria from the anal area.

The best positions for finding his H-spot are either for him to lie on his back with a pillow under his butt and knees raised so you can lie between his thighs and rest your head on one of them, or he can get down on all fours so you can stimulate him from behind. Here are step-by-step instructions on how to find his H-spot and give him oral sex in unison:

1. Insert your finger palm up in a "come here" motion.

2. Once your finger is inside the anus, feel around for a raised nub, which is the prostate gland. Maintain good communication with your partner, and ask him to let you know how it feels using the pleasure scale.

3. Once you've found his H-spot, start tapping it toward the navel in quick succession.

4. Meanwhile, lick his perineum with long, lapping strokes as if you were licking on an ice-cream cone.

Alternatively, you can suck on his testicles, one at a time or both together, while stimulating his H-spot. Another technique is to do the good old-fashioned up-and-down sucking of his penis while stimulating his H-spot.

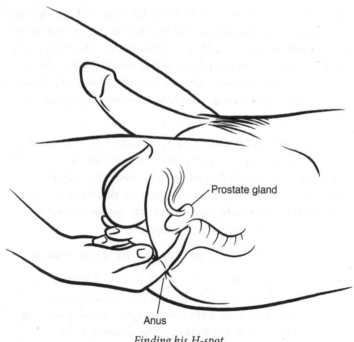

Prostate gland

Anus

Finding his H-spot.

His Outer H-Spot

You can also stimulate his H-spot by rubbing on his perineum, just below his testicles. Remember that men aren't as sensitive to pressure as women, so there's no need to be overly gentle when massaging this area (unless he asks you to lighten up).

1. Start your anal exploration by lightly circling the outside of his anus with your fingers or tongue. You can also try using a small vibrator like the Pocket Rocket.

2. Push your three middle fingers (preferably lubricated), onto the external H-spot, kneading the area as if it were pizza dough. Press in and out, circle one way, then the other, and observe his body language.

3. In the meantime, use your mouth to stimulate his penis by sucking him from the base to the glans in slow motion. Take your time to arouse him to a fever pitch.

4. As his breathing increases, so should your tempo. Don't forget not to change your rhythm before he climaxes unless he asks you to.

Analingus

The most exciting position for a man to receive oral-anal pleasure is on his knees bending over. Here's how to do it:

1. Hold your lover's butt and spread his cheeks slightly apart to expose more of his anus. Because it's a power-packed little bud of erogenous sensitivity, start to lick around the anus with the tip of your tongue clockwise and counterclockwise.

2. Lick up and down over it with the flat of your tongue and side to side over it with the side of your tongue.

3. If your lover's response is positive, and the experience is a turn-on for you, go ahead and penetrate the tip of your tongue inside the anus and push it in and out with quick darting motions.

You can replace your tongue with your finger at any time.

I've mentioned cleanliness and the risks of giving oral sex around the anus in previous chapters. I cannot reiterate the warning enough that analingus can result in contagious STDs; however, it can also be a highly erotic experience. You can use some plastic wrap over the anus or (if you are in a healthy monogamous relationship) take a shower or a bath with your lover so you both feel, look, and taste squeaky clean.

Lots of men love anal play once they're introduced to it by a loving partner. However, some partners are a bit shy in doing it. My advice is: Get over it. If you love your man, give him what he wants.

Have fun!

A

Glossary

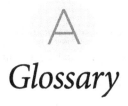

amrita   Female ejaculation fluid.

anal sex   Sexual contact and/or penetration with the anus.

aphrodisiac   A substance that is alleged to stimulate or increase sexual desire.

areola   Pigmented area that surrounds the nipple on the breasts.

butt plug   Sex toy for the anus.

circumcision   The surgical removal of foreskin of the penis.

clap   Gonorrhea.

cleavage fornication   Stimulation of the penis in between the breasts.

climaxing   The point at which orgasm occurs.

clitoral stimulation   To touch the clitoris sexually.

clitoris   A small organ located at the point where the labia minora connect. It plays a vital role in a woman's sexual arousal.

come   To experience orgasm; semen; ejaculation.

consensual sex   Sex as a mutual agreement between two people.

contraception   Birth control.

coronal ridge   The ridge around the head of the penis.

corpus cavernosum   Fills up with blood when stimulated and allows for erection to take place.

corpus spongiosum   A cavity located in the penis that fills with blood during the ejaculatory process.

crura   Part of the clitoris that is made up of two small "wings."

cunniligus   Oral stimulation of a woman's vulva, clitoris, and/or vagina.

deep-throat   A form of oral sex in which the penis is voluntarily taken deeply into the recipient's throat.

delayed ejaculation   Sufferers of delayed or retarded ejaculation find it difficult to ejaculate.

dental dams   Thin squares of latex usually used by dentists but are also used for safer sex practices, especially on women for oral sex.

depilatory cream   Hair removing cream.

dildo   An artificial substitute for an erect penis, made of silicone, rubber, or latex, designed for vaginal or anal insertion for sexual pleasure.

doggie style   A sexual position with man penetrating woman from the rear.

douche   A vaginal rinse.

ejaculation   The expulsion of semen from the penis.

endorphins   A group of peptide hormones found mainly in the brain. Endorphins can reduce the sensation of pain and affect emotions.

epididymis   Coiled tubes located on the side of the testicles that carry new sperm.

erection   Enlargement of the penis when blood flowing to the area causes it to become engorged.

erogenous zones   Areas of the body and skin that respond to sexual stimulation.

fallopian tubes   Two tubes located in the female reproductive system, that lead to the uterus.

fellatio   Oral sexual stimulation of the penis.

female condom   A disposable tube of polyurethane and plastic rings that is inserted into the vagina over the cervix.

female prostatic fluid   Female ejaculation.

fetish   Something such as a material object (shoes) or a non-sexual part of the body (feet) that arouses sexual desire and may become necessary for sexual gratification.

foreplay   Sexual stimulation that happens before intercourse.

foreskin   A fold of thin skin that hangs over the glans of the penis in uncircumcised men.

frenulum   The part of the penis linking the foreskin to the penis, located in the ridge under the glans of the penis.

G-spot First identified by Dr. Ernst Grafenburg and located on the front of the inner upper wall of the vagina, which can result in orgasm when stimulated.

gag reflex The biological reflex that causes someone to feel like they are choking when the back of their throat is stimulated.

genitals The reproductive organs.

glans The head of the penis.

goddess spot *See* G-spot.

hymen A membrane at the entrance to the woman's vagina.

hypoallergenic Minimizes the likelihood of causing an allergic response.

impotence A man's inability to achieve or maintain an erection of sufficient firmness for penetration during intercourse.

intercourse The act of sexual procreation between a man and a woman. Also known as copulation.

Kegel exercises Repeated contractions and release of the pubococcygeus (PC) muscles to strengthen them and increase sexual sensitivity; developed by Dr. Arnold Kegel.

labia majora The outer vaginal lips.

labia minora The inner vaginal lips.

lubricants Solutions that lessen or prevent friction.

masturbation Self-stimulation of one's own genitals for sexual pleasure.

menstruation   The discharge of blood and tissue from the lining of the uterus through the vagina for about three to seven days each month.

missionary position   A sexual position in which the man is on top of the woman.

monogamy   A sexually exclusive relationship, usually as part of a committed relationship.

mons   The soft area above the vagina that is covered with pubic hair.

mons veneris   The pubic hair area.

multiple orgasms   More than one orgasm at a time or in close succession of each other.

mutual masturbation   Sexual contact in which people manually stimulate each other's genitals at the same time.

nipple   The tips of the breasts in men and women.

Nonoxynol-9 spermicide   A spermicide widely used in contraceptive creams, foams, and lubricants.

oral copulation   Sexual stimulation of the male or female genitals using the mouth.

orgasm   Sexual climax, marked by blood flow to the genitals, involuntary rhythmic contraction of the pelvic muscles, and erotic pleasure.

ovaries   Two glands in the female reproductive system that produce eggs during the monthly cycle and hormones that are involved in sexual response development of secondary sex characteristics.

pearl necklace A deposit of semen around the neck.

pelvic floor A series of muscles that form a sling across the opening of the pelvis.

penetration The act of piercing or penetrating something, especially a vagina, with a penis or a tongue.

penis Male reproductive and sex organ.

perineum The area of skin between the genitals and the anus in both men and women.

periurethral sponge *See* G-spot.

plateau A stage of the sexual response cycle in which the excitement maintains a high level prior to climaxing to the orgasm stage.

pornography Written, spoken, or visual material that stimulates sexual feelings.

pre-come *See* pre-ejaculatory fluid.

pre-ejaculatory fluid Fluid secreted by the man's Cowper's glands and discharged from his penis during arousal, prior to ejaculation.

premature ejaculation Ejaculation before the man wants it to occur.

prepuce Protective tissue that covers the clitoris.

prostaglandin-E Hormone that helps men to maintain erection.

prostate exam   Exam that a doctor performs on a man by inserting a gloved lubricated finger into the man's rectum to feel his prostate and detect abnormalities.

prostate gland   A walnut-size gland located below the bladder in a man. It produces the majority of the fluid that combines with sperm and other secretions to make up semen.

prostatectomy   Surgical removal of excess prostate tissue, or in a radical prostatectomy, the removal of the prostate gland.

pubococcygeus (PC) muscles   Pelvic muscles that extend from the pubic bone in the front, around both sides of the sex organs, and back to the tailbone. Control over the PC muscles can enhance sexual response in women and men.

raphe   The seam that runs along the underside of the penis.

rear entry   The sexual position in which the man enters the woman's vagina from behind. Also called "doggie style."

resolution   The final stage of the sexual response cycle, which occurs after orgasm. During this stage, the body returns to the stage it was in prior to excitement.

retarded ejaculation   Sufferers of retarded ejaculation find it difficult to ejaculate. Also known as delayed ejaculation.

rimming   Oral-anal sexual contact.

role-playing   Acting out different roles, often for variety in sexual play.

sadomasochism (S/M or S&M)   A broad term applied to a number of activities such as physical restraining and erotic pain typically involving exchange of power or pain between consenting partners.

saliva   Secretion produced by salivary gland in the mouth.

scrotum   The pouch of skin that hangs below the penis and contains the testes.

semen   Fluid containing sperm that is expelled from the penis during ejaculation. Also called "ejaculate."

seminal vesicles   Two pouches in the male reproductive system, which secrete about 30 percent of the liquid portion of semen.

seminiferous tubes   Tightly coiled tubes located inside each of the testes.

sexual consent   Mutual agreement to have sex.

sexual fantasy   Image of sexual scenario that one creates with one's imagination.

sexual inhibitions   Sexual blocks or suppression.

sexuality   All aspects of one's personality and behaviors that are affected by being male or female.

shaft   Part of penis that extends from the head to beneath the hood.

shrimping   The act of sucking on toes.

sixty-nine   Simultaneous oral sex.

sodomy   Anal or oral penetration.

sperm   The male reproductive cell that is contained in semen, released during ejaculation, and may be united with a woman's egg to cause fertilization and to create life.

spermicide   Products that kill sperm to prevent pregnancy.

sphincter   The muscular ring at the entrance of the anus.

STD   Abbreviation for sexually transmitted disease that can be transmitted through sexual contact.

sterilization   Medical operations performed on men and women to prevent the possibility of reproduction.

taint   Slang term for the perineum.

tea-bagging   Dipping his testicles into your mouth.

testicles (testes)   Two small, oval glands in the scrotum that produce sperm and male hormones.

TriGasm   An orgasm that results from stimulation of three points of pleasure simultaneously.

unilateral copulation   When only one person gives oral sex to another without reciprocation.

unprotected sex   Sex without contraception or protection from STDs.

urethra   The canal that carries urine from the bladder.

uterus   An internal organ of the female reproductive system; also known as the womb.

vagina The muscular passageway that leads from the uterus to the vulva. The area that receives the penis during sexual intercourse.

vagina aerobics Kegel exercises to improve vaginal elasticity.

vaginal discharge Unnatural secretions of the vagina that pertain to some kind of infection.

vas deferens Two narrow tubes that convey sperm to the point where it can mix with the other constituents that make up semen.

vasectomy A surgical method of permanent birth control (sterilization) that involves cutting and tying the vas deferens so a man does not ejaculate sperm yet he still ejaculates semen.

vestibule glands Any of the glands that open into the vestibule of the vagina.

vibrator An electric or battery-operated vibrating device that is often intended for stimulation of the genitals but can be used to massage other parts of the body.

virgin One who has not had sexual intercourse.

vulva Refers to all the external female sexual parts including the mons veneris, the labia majora and minora, the clitoris, the Bartholin's glands, the urethral opening, and vaginal openings.

yeast infection An infection of the mucous membranes caused by the fungus *Candida albicans* inside the vagina.

B

Further Reading and Resources

I believe that even the best lovers can still learn and improve their techniques. The pages that follow list some of the best videos, sex education organizations, and online mail-order sites to make it easy for you to find out more information on your own.

The Best Videos on Oral Sex

The advantage of watching a video on oral sex is that you can observe someone giving it and getting it. You'll be able to emulate exactly what they are doing. Some of the following videos are extremely graphic, so not only will you learn the art of oral sex, but you'll probably get aroused at the same time. And, that's not a bad combination.

Dr. Ava Cadell. *Evolved World Presents The Art of Oral Sex for Couples.* Loveology University, 2011.
This artistically filmed video has three young couples that demonstrate Oral Sex Games and Positions, Oral Sex to Please Her, and Oral Sex to Blow His Mind. You will learn some of the most unique techniques such as The Oral-iental Field Goal, Vertical 69,

and Penis Pilates that will give you the skills to become a great lover. Available at www.loveologyuniversity.com.

Jaiya. *Oral Sex for Couples Series*. New World Sex Education, 2010.
Jaiya is a sassy Sexologist, author of *Red Hot Touch* and producer of many videos, including three volumes of Oral Sex for Couples. Check out all that she has to offer at www.newworld-sexeducation.com.

Tristan Taormino. *Expert Guide to Oral Sex*. Vivid, 2007.
Tristan is a world-class sex educator with a DVD on cunnilingus and a separate one on fellatio where you can watch her lead a group of couples in a hands-on workshop. Tristan's website is www.puckerup.com where you'll find a whole series of sex education videos that include oral and anal sex.

Hartley, Nina. *Nina Hartley's Guide to Better Fellatio*. California: Adam & Eve Productions 1994.
Hall of Fame porn star Nina Hartley teaches and personally demonstrates various fellatio techniques. She gives her own personal insights on arousing your partner, and shares her years of sexual experience.

Hartley, Nina. *Nina Hartley's Guide to Better Cunnilingus*. California: Adam & Eve Productions 1994.
Celebrating a decade of erotic performing, Nina Hartley wrote and directed this video for everyone interested in expanding their sexual horizon and pleasing their mate orally.

Sinclair Intimacy Institute. *Better Oral Sex Techniques*. Sinclair Intimacy Institute, 1997.
The Sinclair Institute has released a guide to cunnilingus and fellatio as part of their series on how-to tapes. It features sex

experts Dr. Marty Klein and Dr. Diana Wiley who introduce basic techniques that can help couples master cunnilingus and fellatio. Couples demonstrate oral sex on each other, and viewers can discover new ways to enjoy oral delights.

Dodson, Betty. *Betty Dodson's Celebrating Orgasm.* Pacific Media Entertainment, 2000.
This video is a great teaching tool for women and those who love them. Betty Dodson personally guides women on how to orgasm and how to get in touch with themselves sexually. The result is "Seven Techniques for Achieving Orgasmic Ecstasy, the foundation of Celebrating Orgasm."

Perry, Dr. Michael. *Sexual Secrets a Sex Surrogate's Guide to Great Lovemaking.* BCI Eclipse Company, 1994.
Sex therapist Dr. Michael Perry has produced a series of sex educational videos titled *The Intimacy Guide for Couples.* In this video, you'll see a sex surrogate teach some hot techniques on giving and getting oral sex. Other lessons include sex talk, sexual positions, and intercourse.

Sex Education and Therapy

Whether you're interested in finding out the answer to a pressing sex question, looking for a sex therapist in your neighborhood, or interested in becoming a sexologist yourself, the list of sex education resources here will lead you in the right direction.

Loveology University
Loveology University offers an online Certified Love Coaching Program and a Master Sexpert Certification. You will also find a variety of videos, audios, slideshow courses, and e-books on love,

romance, relationships, intimacy, and sexuality at
www.loveologyuniversity.com.

The Institute for Advanced Study of Human Sexuality

This graduate school is one of the few in the world approved
to train clinical sexologists. They also have an impressive sex
museum where you can trace the history of sex. For more information on their degrees, you can call 415-928-1133 or go to their
website at www.iashs.edu.

Sexuality Information and Education Council of the United States (SIECUS)

SIECUS is a national nonprofit organization that affirms that
sexuality is a natural and healthy part of living. It develops, col-
lects, and circulates information on sex education and advocates
the right of individuals to make responsible sexual choices. For
more information call 212-819-9770 or visit www.siecus.org.

The American Association of Sex Educators, Counselors, and Therapists (AASECT)

AASECT is a nonprofit, interdisciplinary professional organization. If you are looking for a sex educator, sexologist, sex
counselor, or sex therapist, AASECT can help you find one they
have certified in your area. Members of AASECT share an inter-
est in promoting understanding of human sexuality and healthy
sexual behavior. Call 804-644-3288, or go to www.aasect.org.

American Association of Marriage and Family Therapists (AAMFT)

The AAMFT Directory will assist you in locating a marriage and
family therapist in your area. The listed therapists are clinical
members of the American Association for Marriage and Family
Therapy. The directory provides information on the therapist's

office locations and availability, practice description, education, professional licenses, health plan participation, achievements and awards, and languages spoken. Call 202-452-0109, or visit www.aamft.org.

Mail-Order and Online Stores

Lots of people feel uncomfortable going to a sex shop, especially if they live in a small town where everyone knows each other. Now there's a better way to purchase your sex toys and sensual lingerie. It's anonymous, and it's easy.

Adam and Eve Catalog
This is one of the largest catalogs in the adult industry. You'll find the latest sex toys, sex education videos, adult DVDs, safer sex supplies, and lingerie. Call 1-800-274-0333 or go to their website at www.adameve.com.

Good Vibrations
This is a retail store located in San Francisco that has a catalog and a website where you can find information on sexual health, pleasure, and current events. You can also purchase sex toys, sex education, erotic and how-to books, and adult videos. Call 1-800-289-8423, or visit www.goodvibes.com.

Xandria Collection
For more than 30 years, the Xandria Collection has been one of America's top resources for sex toys, lingerie, and sex education. On their website, you can ask questions, learn about the history of sex, read jokes, or buy some sexy ecards. Call 1-800-242-2823 or go to www.xandria.com.

Toys in Babeland

This is a sex toy store run by women whose mission is to promote and celebrate sexual vitality by providing an honest, open, and fun environment. They not only offer the latest sex gadgets, but lingerie, lotions, and safer sex supplies, and you can even join one of their workshops. Call 1-800-658-9119, or check them out at www.toysinbabeland.com.

The publisher would like to thank Amory Abbott for the illustrations in this book.